NUCLEAR ENERGY SIMPLIFIED

AN OVERVIEW OF THE NUCLEAR TECHNOLOGY
OF REACTORS, SPACE AND MEDICINE

By

FRANK L. BOUQUET

Physicist A.A., B.A., M.A.

Systems Co.

ISBN 1-56216-073-7(Hardcover) $55
ISBN 1-56216-074-5(Paper) $35

            Library of Congress Cataloging-in-Publication Data

Bouquet, Frank L.
    Nuclear energy simplified : an overview of the nuclear technology
of reactors, space, and medicine / by Frank L. Bouquet. -- Original
ed.
        p.   cm.
    Includes bibliographical references and indexes.
    ISBN 1-56216-073-7 : $55.00. -- ISBN 1-56216-074-5 (pbk.) : $35.00
    1. Nuclear energy. 2. Nuclear reactors. 3. Nuclear propulsion.
4. Nuclear medicine.   I. Title.
TK9145.B59   1992
621.48--dc20   92-6091
                                                              CIP

STATEMENT OF CONFIDENTIALITY

PREFACE

It has been almost a century since Roentgen discovered radioactivity in 1895. During the past 50 years, a tremendous amount of nuclear technology has been developed. Much of it is a complete mystery to many not in the field.

Actually, the basic principles of nuclear energy are simple-only the technical details are complex.

It is the purpose of this book to present an up-to-date status of atomic and nuclear technology for the layperson or the technical specialist just entering the field. Special care is taken to define the many technical terms because the jargon is a major hurdle to understanding.

A glossary is included as well as References and Bibliography for those who wish to delve further.

This book is an outgrowth of lectures given to engineers at the Lockheed Astronautical Systems Company, namely Science Seminar, Fundamentals of Nuclear Radiation and Physics of Nuclear Propulsion. Because I have followed the developments in the last 45 years in the areas of nuclear reactors, space technology and nuclear medicine, I feel qualified to write this book at this time. My 14 years as a member of the NASA team at the Jet Propulsion Laboratory was a growth period that gave me new insights to space technology.

The field of nuclear energy is by no means closed. Scientists are at work in many new areas, including cold fusion, hot fusion and new particle discoveries. New types of commercial power reactors are being developed. Third world countries are scrambling to build nuclear reactors and destructive weapons. All the time, we are experiencing ground level radiation from the sun, cosmic rays and medical exposures.

This book casts all these phenomena into understandable terms.

CONTENTS

Chapter 1

INTRODUCTION

Over the last century, much technology has evolved using the nucleus and atomic shells of the atom.

It all started with the discovery of radioactivity in 1895 by wilhelm Roengten. Since then, the technology has continued by leaps and bounds.

Nuclear technology covers lots of smaller, specialized technologies. Some of these are shown in Figure 1-1.

The various areas are vast so just the top of the iceberg is treated in this book. It is hoped that it will be useful in imparting a basic understanding and stimulating the student to research further.

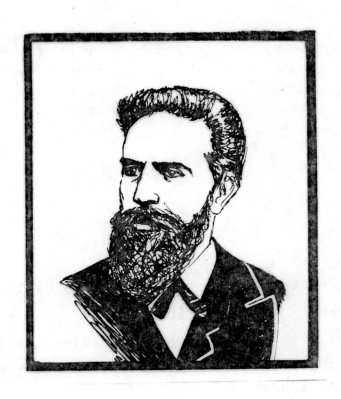

WILLIAM CONRAD RÖNTGEN

(1845-1923)

Dr. Röntgen, or Roentgen, was a German physicist who won the 1901 Nobel Prize for his discovery of X-rays.

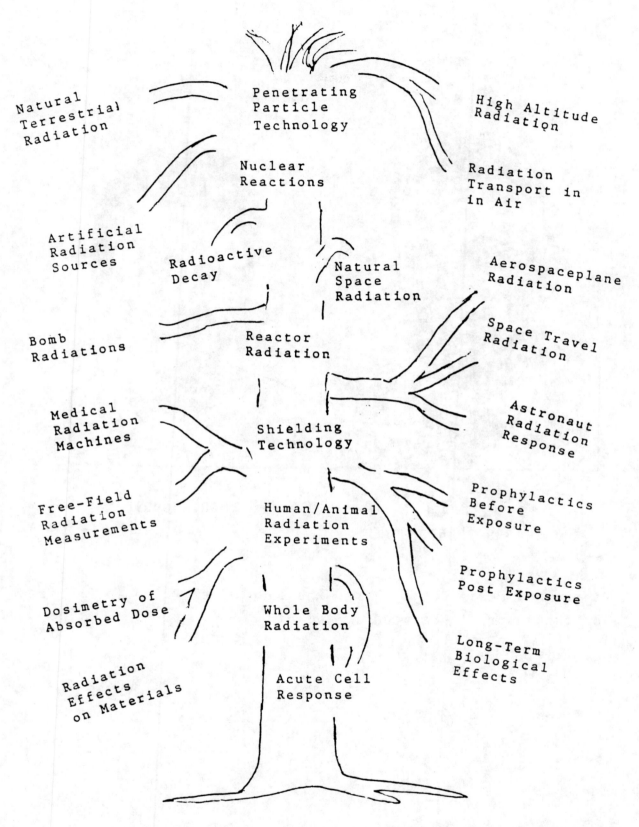

Natural Terrestrial Radiation

Penetrating Particle Technology

High Altitude Radiation

Nuclear Reactions

Radiation Transport in in Air

Artificial Radiation Sources

Radioactive Decay

Natural Space Radiation

Aerospaceplane Radiation

Bomb Radiations

Reactor Radiation

Space Travel Radiation

Medical Radiation Machines

Shielding Technology

Astronaut Radiation Response

Free-Field Radiation Measurements

Human/Animal Radiation Experiments

Prophylactics Before Exposure

Dosimetry of Absorbed Dose

Prophylactics Post Exposure

Radiation Effects on Materials

Whole Body Radiation

Long-Term Biological Effects

Acute Cell Response

Figure 1-1 The Nuclear Energy Technology Tree

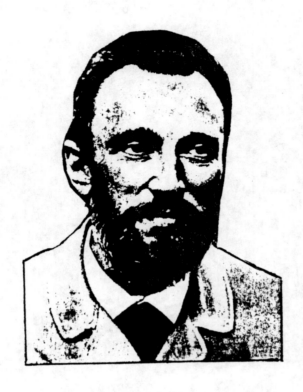

PIERRE CURIE
(1859-1906)

MARIE CURIE

Pierre and Marie Curie shared the 1903 Nobel Prize in Physics for their work in radioactivity.

TYPES OF NUCLEAR ENERGY

There are basically two types of nuclear energy, namely:

o Fission Energy
  This form of energy results from the breaking up of atoms and usually occurs with low energy particles.

o Fusion Energy
  This form of energy takes very high energy particles to initiate it. It is the fusing together of two (or more) atoms to make one more compact atom.

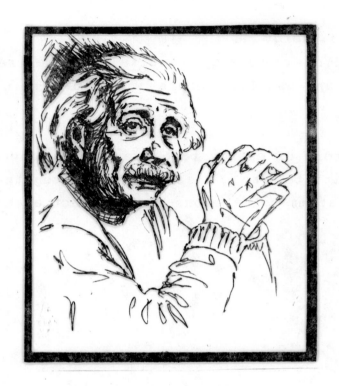

DR. ALBERT EINSTEIN

(1879-1955)

Dr. Albert Einstein discovered the Special Theory of Relativity
(1905) and the General Theory of Relativity(1915).

FISSION ENERGY

Fission heat occurs due to the breakup of heavy elements, such as uranium and plutonium.

Heat

Heavy element

~ ½ atom

~ ½ atom

Neutron

Electromagnetic radiation, X-rays

particles

The heavy element breaks up into two smaller atoms of approximately one-half of the original atom. Energy is released in the process along with radiations.

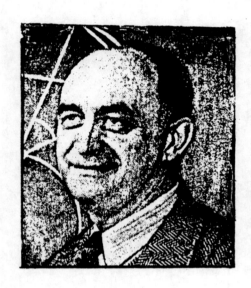

Dr. Enrico Fermi

(1901-1954)

Dr. Enrico Fermi, an Italian-born physicist, discovered the neutron and supervised the first nuclear chain reaction at the University of Chicago, Illinois.

In 1954, the U.S. Atomic Energy Commission awarded him a $25,000 award in recognition of his work on the atomic bomb.

A TYPICAL COMMERCIAL
NUCLEAR REACTOR

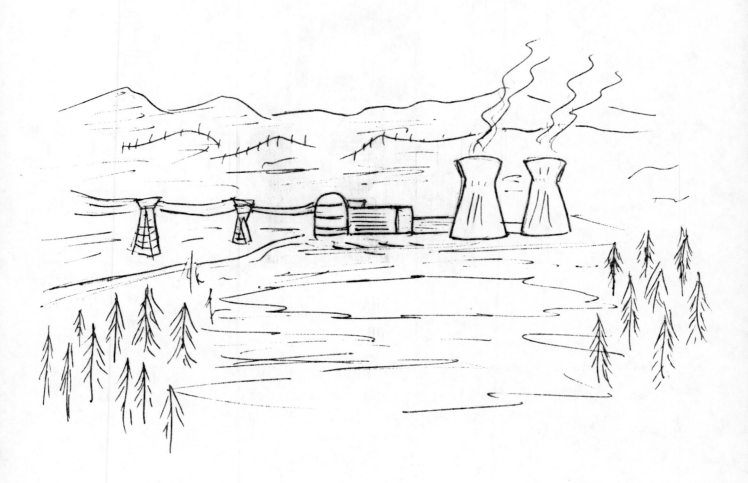

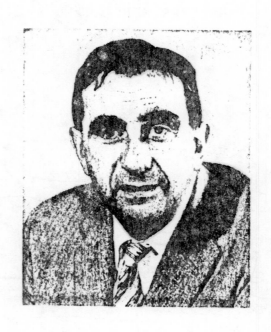

DR. EDWARD TELLER

(1908 -   )

Dr. Edward Teller, a nuclear physicist, participated in the
production of the first nuclear chain reaction and the first
atomic bomb. He has been referred to as "The Father of the
Hydrogen Bomb."

FUSION ENERGY

Another type of nuclear energy is the coming together of small particles to produce one larger particle. This is the type of reaction that occurs in the sun and can be produced in the laboratory.

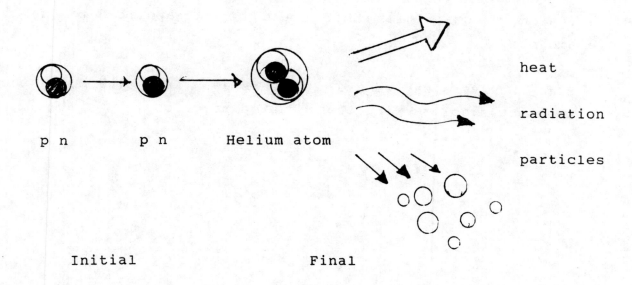

Because it is more efficient in nature to have a compact structure, the excess energy (binding energy) is released as heat.

FUSION ENERGY (Cont.)

Theoretically, fusion processes may occur at room temperature. This is called "cold fusion" because it should not take extremely high particle impact energies.

Although articles concerning it have appeared over the last 30 years, recent experiments have failed to produce cold fusion in quantities that could be extrapolated to useful amounts.

Some observers say we are 20 years away from overcoming the inherent problems with these fusion reactions.

EXPERIMENTAL FUSION DEVICE

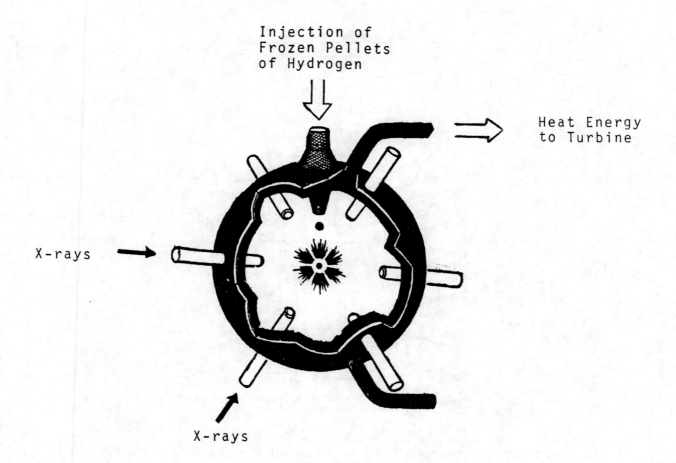

Through the use of very short, high
energy X-rays, extremely high temperatures
are achieved in the center of the cavity.

THERMONUCLEAR REACTOR
Reference 46.

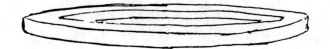

Vertical Field
Magnet

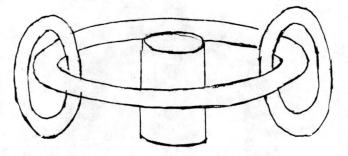

Toroidal Field
Magnet

Central Transformer
Magnet

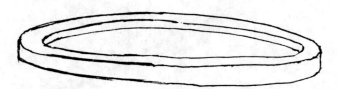

This experimental fusion reactor is 13 years away from
completion. It is a Takamak Fusion Reactor.

- o It relies on the deuterium-tritium reaction.
- o It has a first-wall problem as do other fusion
     devices. The diagnostic and other instruments are
     located in a shielding wall that undergoes rapid
     degradation. In some designs, it is replaced freq-
     uently.
- o The vertical magnets keep the plasma in equilibium.
- o The toroidal magnets act as a sleeve to confine the
     plasma.

SUMMARY

Over the last century, we have seen the identification of a vast new technology that uses the atomic and nuclear properties of the atom.

While the fission process has been put to commerical use, the fusion process has not. Over the next century we may practical applications of fusion.

Both of these processes work using tiny particles. These are treated in the next section.

BLANK PAGE

Chapter 2

PARTICLES

In this chapter, the properties of the various nuclear particles are presented.

There are over 100 known nuclear particles with more being discovered every day. However, in practical experience, such as around a nuclear reactor, plain types of particles are encountered, i.e., neutrons and protons.

Many of the particles take high energies to make them, hence the research on the big cyclotrons and linacs.

Nonetheless, this chapter should serve as an introduction to the state-of-the-art in particle technology.

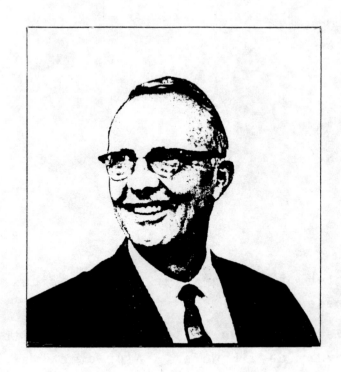

DR. LUIS WALTER ALVAREZ

(1911-1988)

Dr. Alvarez, a professor at the University of California, won the Nobel Prize in Physics in 1968 for his work in high energy cosmic rays and particle physics.

Table 2-1

PARTICLE ROUNDUP

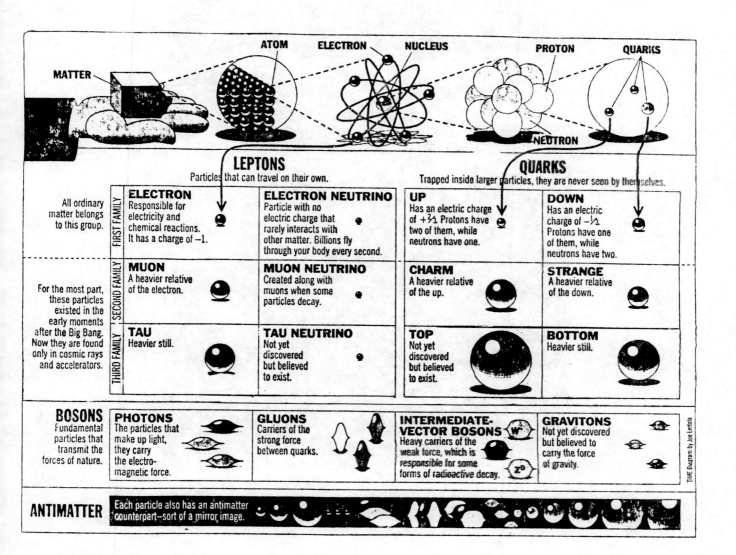

Courtesy Time Magazine, April 16, 1990.

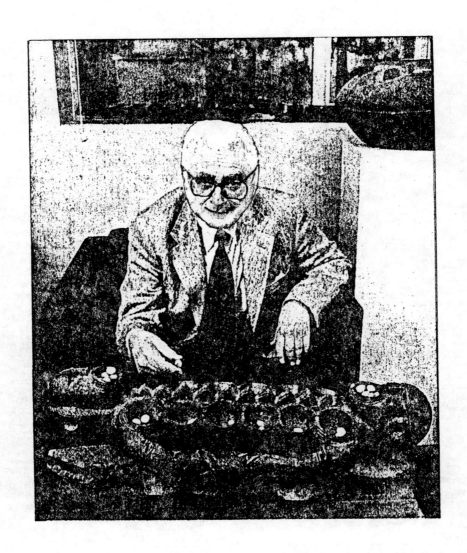

DR. MURRAY GELL-MANN

Dr. Murray Gell-Mann, a professor at the California Institute of Technology, received the Nobel Prize for his work in sub-atomic particles, including the discovery of the quark.

Table 2-2

The Elementary Particles

Class	Name	Particle	Antiparticle	Mass, m_e	Spin	Mean lifetime, sec	Lepton number L	Baryon number B	Strangeness number S
Photon	photon	γ	(γ)	0	1	stable	0	0	0
Leptons	neutrino	ν, ν_μ	$\bar{\nu}, \bar{\nu}_\mu$	0	½	stable	+1	0	0
	electron	e^-	e^+	1	½	stable	+1	0	0
	μ meson	μ^-	μ^+	207	½	2.22×10^{-6}	+1	0	-1
Mesons	π meson	π^+	π^-	273	0	2.54×10^{-8}	0	0	0
		π^0	(π^0)	264	0	2.3×10^{-16}	0	0	0
	K meson	K^+	K^-	967	0	1.22×10^{-8}	0	0	+1
		K^0	$\bar{K}^0$	967	0	$10^{-10}, 6 \times 10^{-8}$	0	0	+1
Baryons	proton	p^+	$\bar{p}^-$	1,836	½	stable	0	+1	0
	neutron	n^0	$\bar{n}^0$	1,839	½	1.11×10^3	0	+1	0
	Λ hyperon	Λ^0	$\bar{\Lambda}^0$	2,182	½	2.5×10^{-10}	0	+1	-1
	Σ hyperon	Σ^+	$\bar{\Sigma}^-$	2,328	½	0.8×10^{-10}	0	+1	-1
		Σ^-	$\bar{\Sigma}^-$	2,343	½	1.6×10^{-10}	0	+1	-1
		Σ^0	$\bar{\Sigma}^0$	2,341	½	$<10^{-11}$	0	+1	-1
Baryons	Ξ hyperon	Ξ^-	$\bar{\Xi}^-$	2,583	½	1.3×10^{-10}	0	+1	-2
		Ξ^0	$\bar{\Xi}^0$	2,571	½	1.5×10^{-10}	0	+1	-2

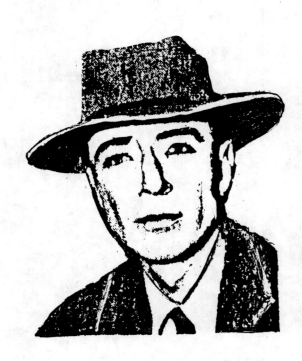

Dr. J. ROBERT OPPENHEIMER

(1904-1967)

Dr. Oppenheimer, a consultant to the U.S. Atomic Energy Commission, was responsible for directing the Los Alamos National
Laboratory in New Mexico during World War II. Later he taught
physics at the University of California(Berkeley) and   the
California Institute of Technology.

RELATIVE SIZES OF ATOMS

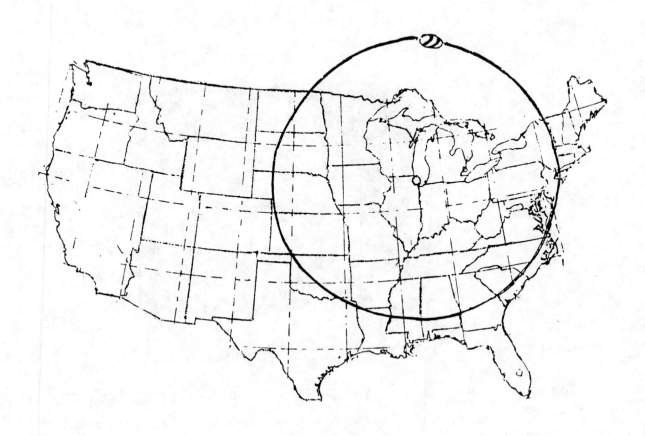

Figure 2-1

It is difficult to imagine the openness of atoms. As an illustration, if the nucleus is represented as a cantalope centered in Chicago, the electron is a watermelon orbiting at a distance of New York City!

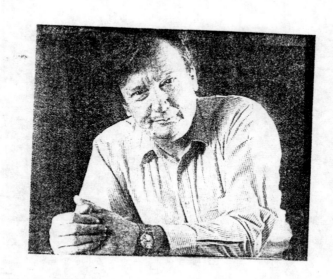

DR. CARLO RUBBIA

Dr. Carlo Rubbia is responsible for the discovery of subatomic
particles, especially the W and Z particles. He shared   the
Nobel Prize in Physics for his work.

COMPOSITION OF THE NUCLEI OF ATOMS

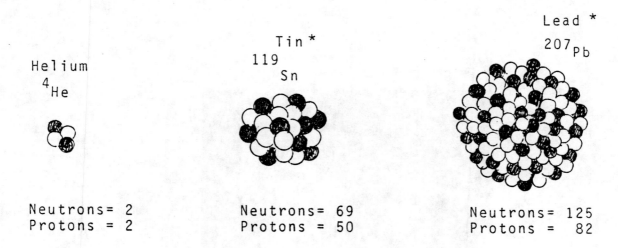

Helium
^{4}He

Neutrons= 2
Protons = 2

Tin *
119
Sn

Neutrons= 69
Protons = 50

Lead *
^{207}Pb

Neutrons= 125
Protons = 82

Each nucleus may be stable with a number
of isotopes, perhaps one to 10, each with
the same number of protons.

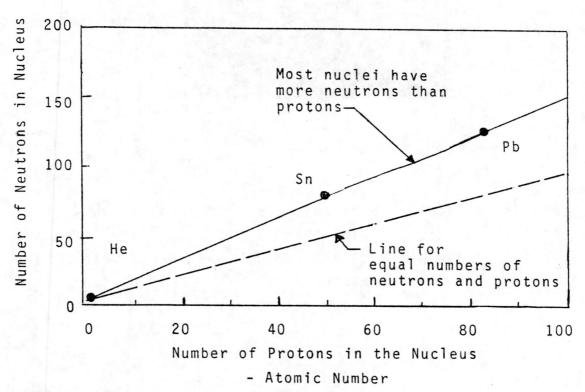

Figure 2-2

* Actually, there are four
separate isotopes of this
same atomic number that are
stable.

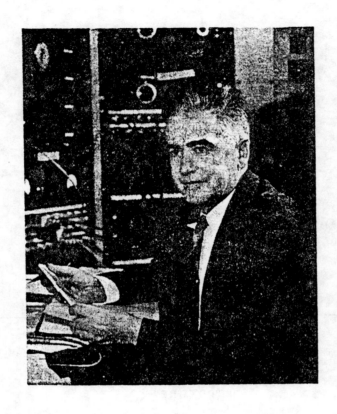

DR. EMILIO(Gino) SEGRÈ

Dr. Segrè was an Italian-born physicist who received the Nobel Prize in 1955 for his work in the discovery of antimatter (negatively-charged protons). The prize was shared with his colleague, Dr. Owen Chamberlain.

Table 2-3

Energy Ranges of Typical Radiations

Radiation	Typical Range
Alpha Particles	Up to 7 MeV
Beta Particles	Up to 5 MeV
Gamma Rays from Nuclear Fission Decay	Up to 3 MeV
Gamma Rays from Fission	Up to 20 MeV
Positrons	Up to 3 MeV
Protons	Depends upon the cyclotron or accelerator energy range typically 0- 200 MeV
Electrons	Depends upon the type of accelerator, typically up to 20 BeV
Neutrons	
Fast	Greater than 0.1 MeV
Intermediate	Greater than thermal energy (0.025 eV) to 0.1 MeV
Thermal	About 0.025 eV

Table 2-4

Gamma Ray Interactions

Interaction Process	Energy of Gamma Ray	Primary Effect
Photoelectric	Less than 1.0 MeV	Direct Absorption
Compton Process	1- 5 MeV	Slowing down and scattering with secondary electrons generated
Pair Production	Greater than 5 MeV	Formation of electrons and positrons.

To obtain the absorbed dose in the material, further analysis (or access to test data) is needed concerning the specific mass absorption coefficient for the particular type of material under consideration.

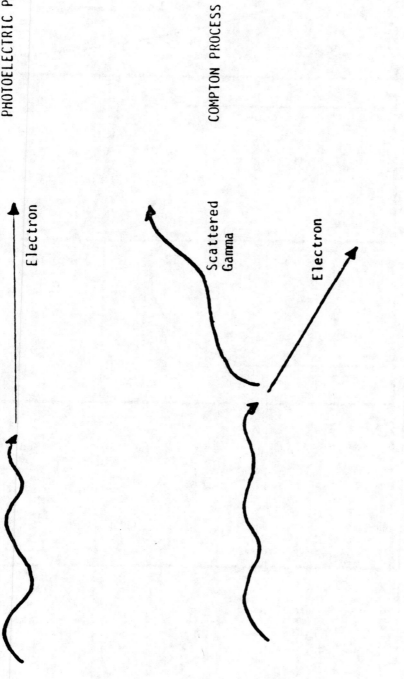

PHOTOELECTRIC PROCESS

Electron

COMPTON PROCESS

Scattered
Gamma

Electron

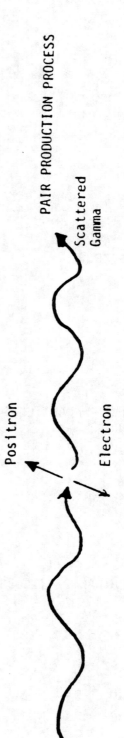

PAIR PRODUCTION PROCESS

Scattered
Gamma

Positron

Electron

2-13

Figure 2-3   Primary Gamma Ray Interactions with Materials

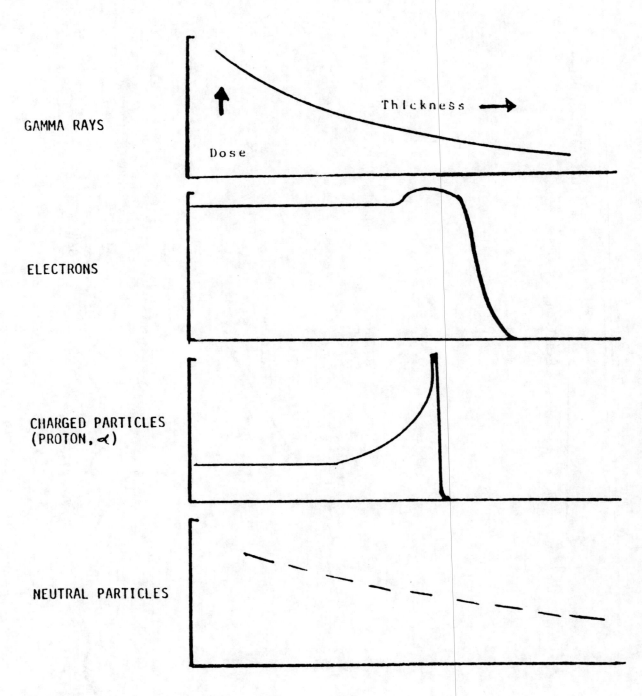

Figure 2-4   Comparison of Dose
versus Thickness

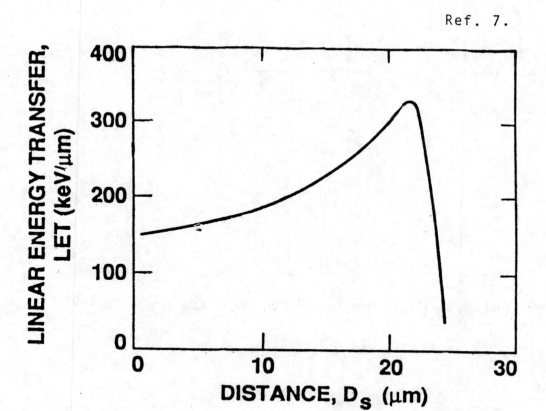

Figure 2-5

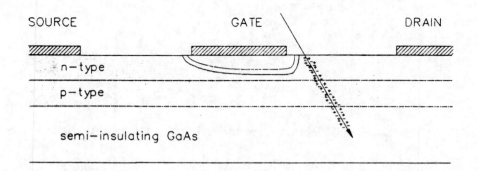

Schematic diagram of an ion track in a 1 μm gate length depletion-mode GaAs MESFET

Figure 2-6

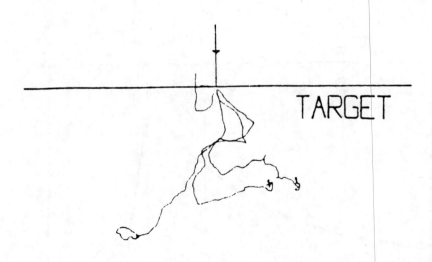

Computer plot showing five electron trajectories in a Cu target with a 20 keV incident beam normal to the surface.

Figure 2-7

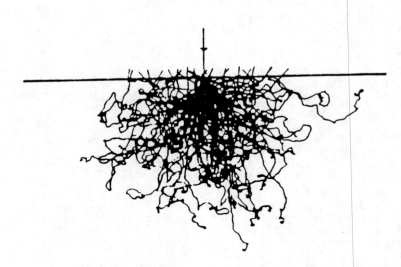

Monte Carlo results for 100 electron trajectories in a Cu target with 20 keV incident electron energy.[7]

Figure 2-8

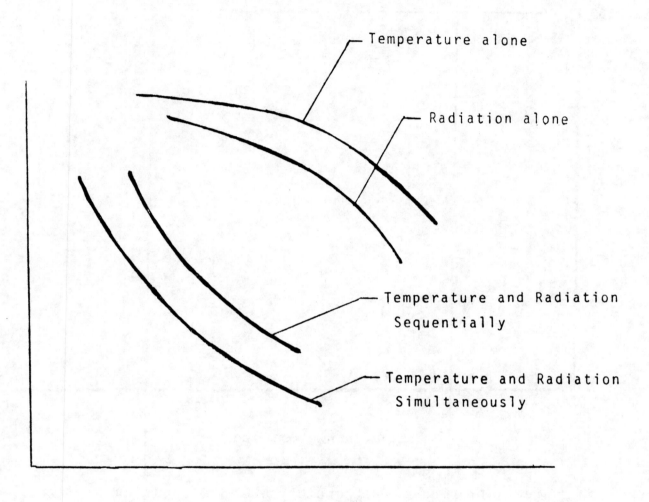

Figure 2-9   Typical Effects of Temperature and
Radiation Acting on a Material

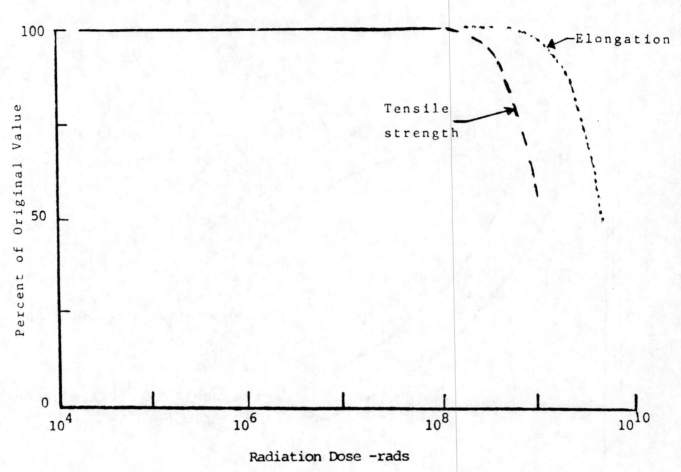

Category: Insulator

Material: Polyimide, Kapton H-Film

Figure 2-10   Tensile Strength vs. and Elongation
vs. Radiation Dose.

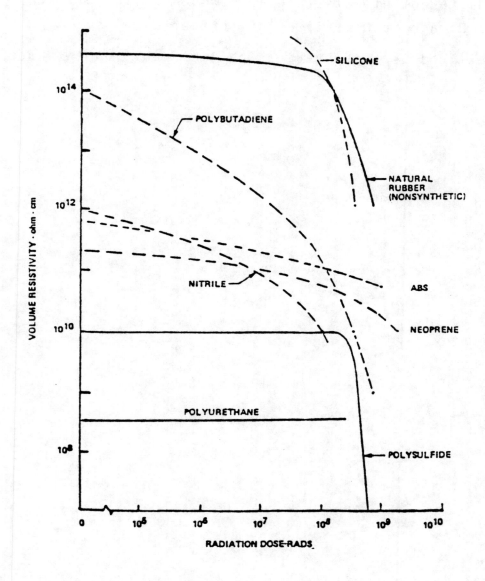

Figure 2-11   Volume Resistivity vs Radiation
             Dose for Selected Elastomers.

2-19

Particles(Cont.)

In this chapter, we have seen that a wide variety of particles exist in nature.

Each has different properties and operate over different ener specific energy ranges. As they interact with matter, they produce different effects that are frequently complicated. See Radiation Damage in Materials for further details.

In the next chapter, the various particle environments are treated.

Chapter 3

ENVIRONMENTS

The particles treated in the last chapter are capable of producing important environments on both Earth and in in space.

Some of the characteristics of these environments are given in this chapter.

NATURAL BACKGROUND RADIATION

No matter where we are, we are exposed to penetrating nuclear radiation everyday.

The sources of this radiation vary widely with location and time. Fortunately the radiation is very low level and the biological effects are small.

This radiation can be divided into two types:
- o Steady state radiation
  - Examples are the cosmic rays and radiation coming from the earth beneath us. Both vary widely with location on the earth. (Ref. 27)
- o Transient radiation
  - Examples are:
  Giant air bursts of cosmic rays that hit the top of the atmosphere every day and produce fast moving secondaries at sea level.

  Low level radiation being emitted from the foods we eat or the people we are near. (Ref. 29)

HIGH ALTITUDE RADIATION

People who live in high altitudes or fly in aircraft receive higher radiation than those at lower altitudes. Fortunately, this radiation is quite small, maybe a factor of two higher in most cases. Intermittent transient radiation at higher levels can be encountered when solar sunspot activity occurs.

The plasma and penetrating solar cosmic rays are infrequent.

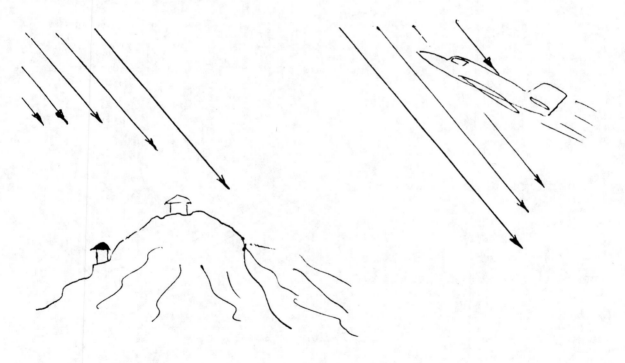

High Altitude   Airplane Altitude

Figure 3-2 Two Regions of High Altitude Radiation
in the Atmosphere.

NUCLEAR RADIATION FROM THE
SUN AND SPACE

We are exposed to penetrating nuclear particles generated by the sun and galaxies. Fortunately, the intensities are low and much is absorbed by the earth's atmosphere of 30 grams per square centimeter. This is equivalent to 30 feet of concrete.

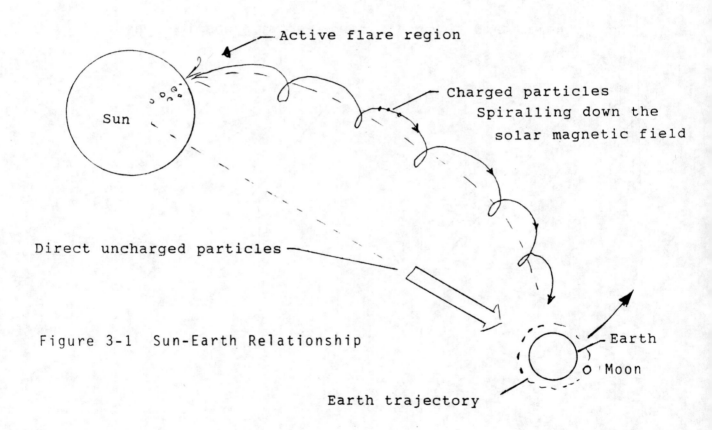

Figure 3-1 Sun-Earth Relationship

Nonetheless, some particles penetrate down to sea level and on into the deepest mines, such as neutrinos.

Their effects are small (Ref. 27).

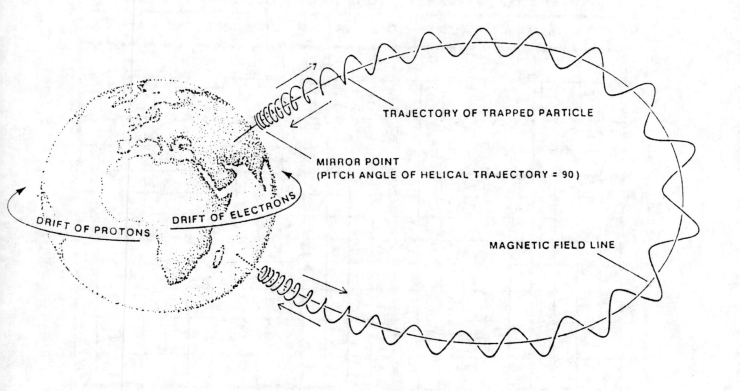

Figure 3-3

Motions of the Particles (Protons and Electrons)
Trapped in the Earth's Magnetic Field.

Ref. 5.

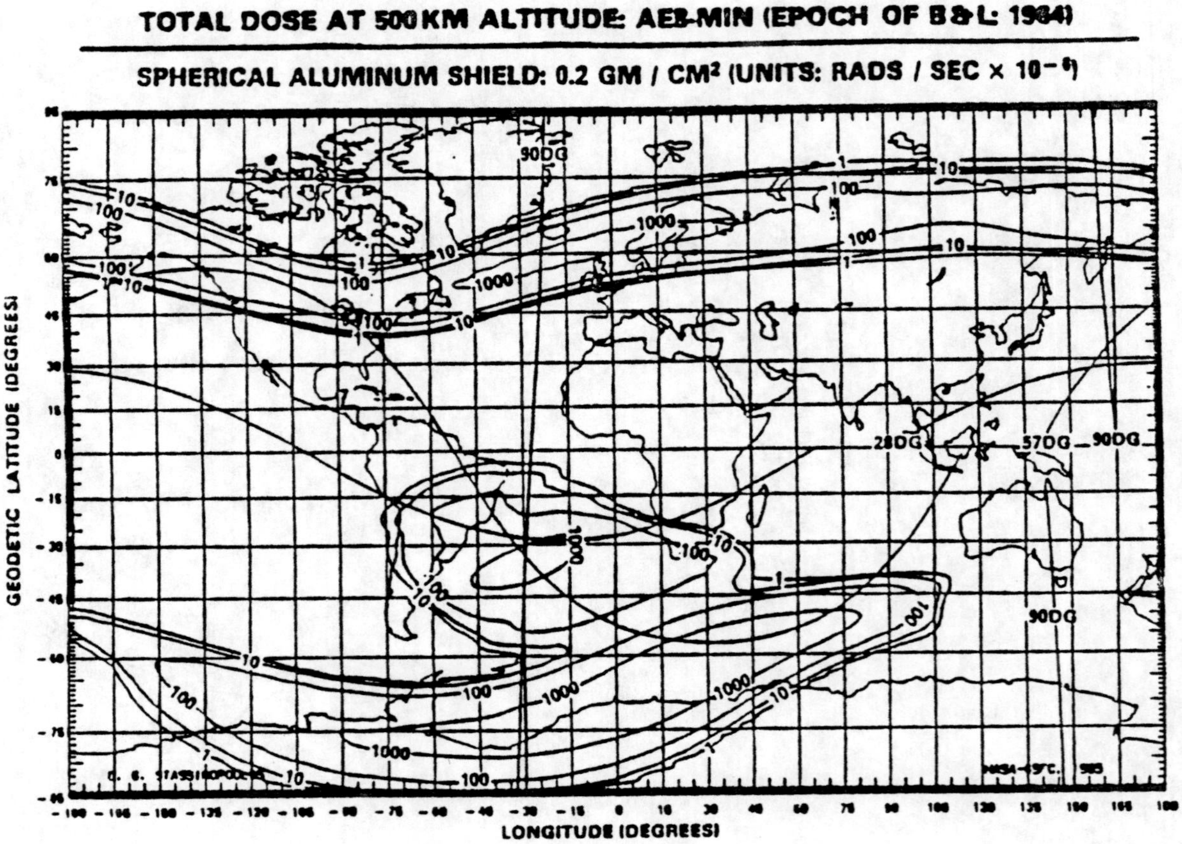
TOTAL DOSE AT 500KM ALTITUDE: AE8-MIN (EPOCH OF B&L: 1964)
SPHERICAL ALUMINUM SHIELD: 0.2 GM / CM² (UNITS: RADS / SEC x 10⁻⁶)
GEODETIC LATITUDE (DEGREES)
LONGITUDE (DEGREES)
90DG
28DG
57DG

Figure 3-4 A World Contour of the Dose Received While Orbiting the Earth. The Dose is Behind o.2 Grams/cm^2 Shield. High Regions Are Seen Over the North and South and Over the South Atlantic Anomaly.

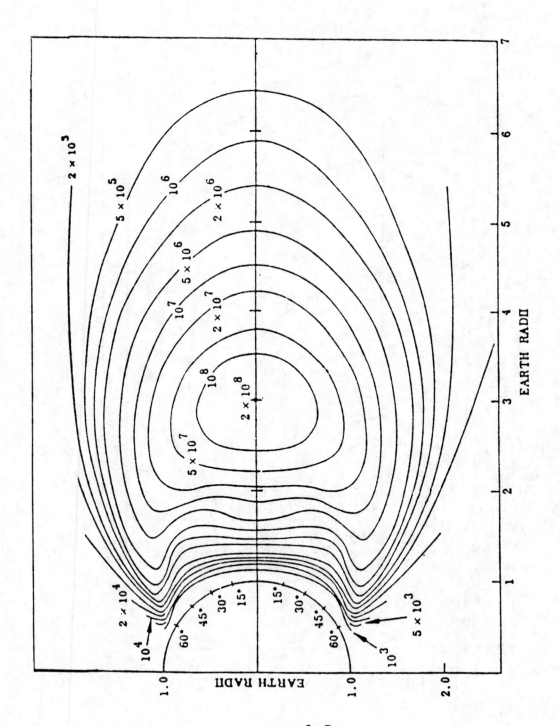

Figure 3-5 Locations of the Earth's Trapped Protons.

3-7

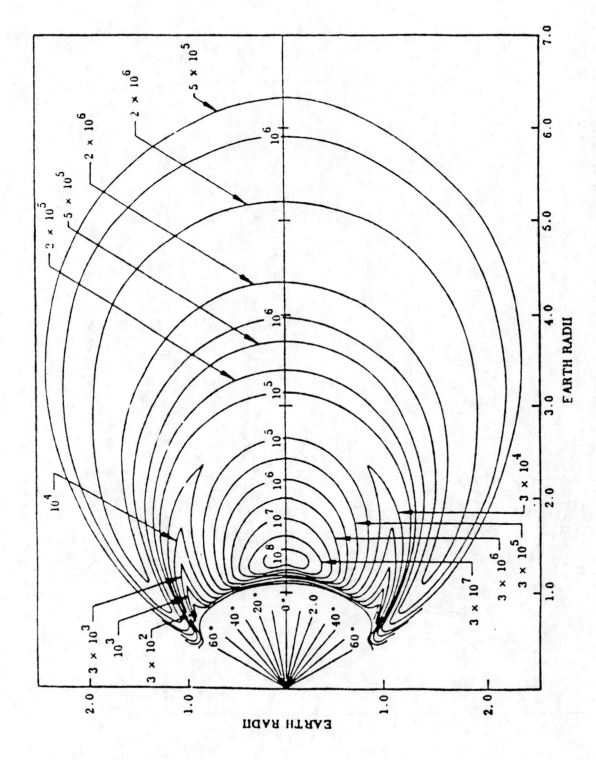

Figure 3-6 Locations of the Earth's Trapped Protons.

3-8

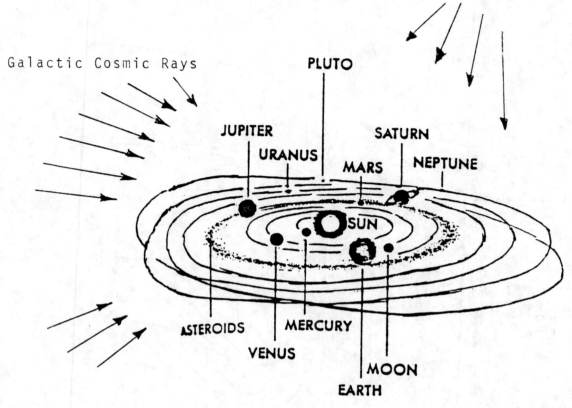

Galactic Cosmic Rays

PLUTO

JUPITER
URANUS
MARS
SATURN
NEPTUNE

SUN

ASTEROIDS
MERCURY
VENUS
MOON
EARTH

Ref. 26.

Figure 3-7   View of Our Solar System. The Sun is the Source
of Many of the Particles Hitting the Top of Our
Atmosphere. The Earth, Jupiter, Saturn and and
Venus Are Known to Have Radition Belts.

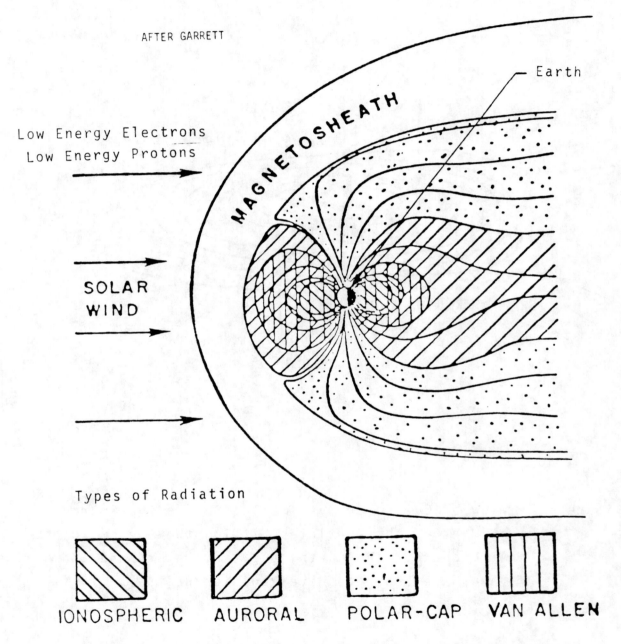

AFTER GARRETT

Low Energy Electrons
Low Energy Protons

MAGNETOSHEATH

Earth

SOLAR
WIND

Types of Radiation

IONOSPHERIC   AURORAL   POLAR-CAP   VAN ALLEN

Figure 3-8 The Solar Wind-Earth Relationship

The particles found in space are dynamic. They change
with time and location.

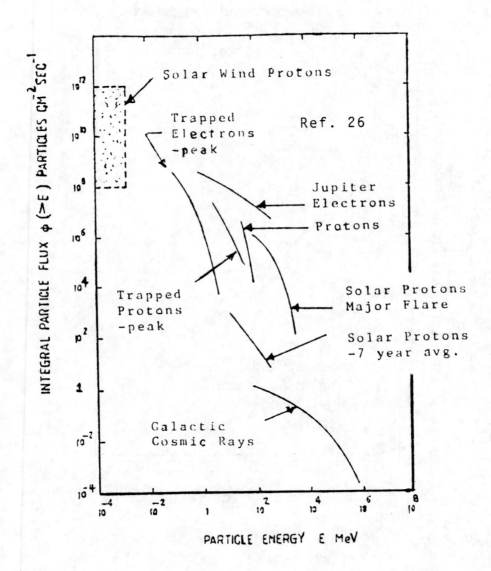

Figure 3-9   Summary of the Various Radiations in
              Space.   The Total Number of Particles
              Intercepted vs. Energy.

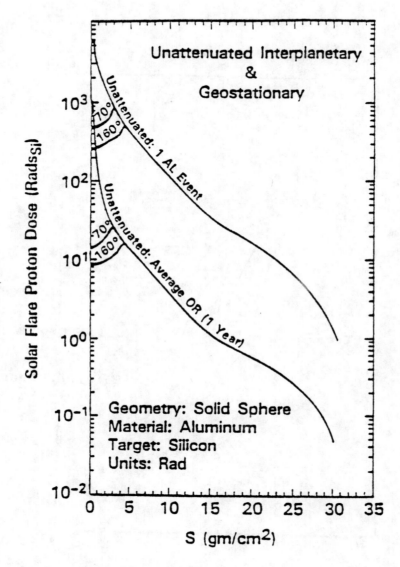

Figure 3-10 The Radiation(Dose) Received in a
Silicon Detector in Space behind
Increasing Thicknesses of Aluminum(S).

Chapter 4

TERRESTRIAL RADIATION

Within the Earth's atmosphere, we have very low level radiation that increases with altitude. In 1958, the Van Allen
radiation belts that encircle the Earth were discovered.

Radition comes from many sources:

- o The ground because dirt contains minute amounts
  of radioactive materials. In some regions,
  a radioactive gas, radon, diffuses up from the
  Earth.
- o Solar cosmic rays sometimes reach the surface of
  of the Earth and the Cosmic Galactic rays do
  quite frequently. Fortunately, they are very
  weak.
- o Machines, such as medical devices.
- o Radioactive sources
- o Aircraft or spacecraft that travel near or beyond the atmosphere of the Earth may be exposed to higher radiation.

4-1

In this chapter, some of the more important radiation
sources are given.

NUCLEAR REACTORS

Nuclear reactors use uranium to produce power. Heat from the fissioning process is used to heat water into steam. The steam drives a generator to produce electricity. Of course, this latter component is not present in research reactors where the effects of radiation on materials are investigated.

Reactors can be classified into the following categories:

o Research reactors.

o Electric Power Stationary Reactors.

o Mobile nuclear reactors, such as used to propel sub-marines and surface ships.

All three work on the same principles. A combination radiation and heat shielding is needed to isolate the reactors from personnel and sensitive equipment.

NUCLEAR REACTOR SYSTEM

A Typical Reactor System

To Turbine

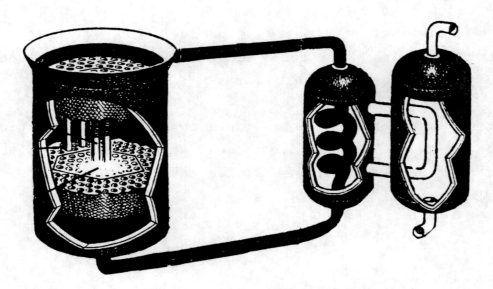

Heat Exchanger

Reactor Core
with Control Rods

Table 4-1

World Nuclear Power*

The United States leads the world in the amount of nuclear power produced. This is shown in the Table along with countries producing lesser amounts.

Country	Amount of Nuclear Power Produced (1988)
U.S.	$526,900 \times 10^{6}$ Kilowatt-hours
France	260,200
USSR	204,000
Japan	163,100
West Germany	137,300
Canada	78,200
Sweden	65,600
Great Britain	55,600
Spain	48,300
Belgium	40,000

* Source: World Book Encyclopedia, Vol. 14, 1991.

NUCLEAR-POWERED VEHICLES

Many studies have been performed to develop long-lived propulsion units.

Examples are:

Trains

Cars

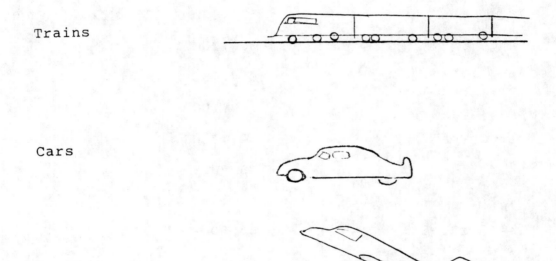

Planes

Advantages are low-pollution, high power density and long lives.

So far, they have not been feasible due to the heavy shielding requirements and the radioactive hazards due to accidents.

NUCLEAR POWERED SATELLITES

Two types of nuclear applications have been used on satellites.
- o Electrical Power Systems
- o Radioactive Heaters

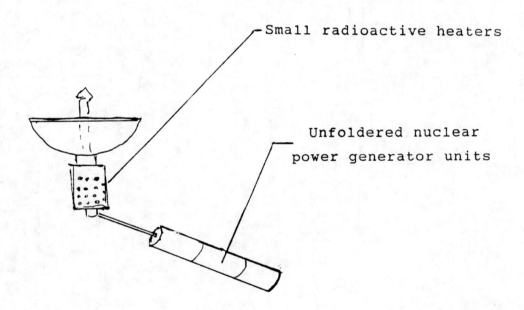

Figure 4-2   Sketch of Nuclear Power on Satellite

Specially designed nuclear power modules are used. Compositions are typically either uranium or plutonium. The generator units supply constant power for long-lived missions. The small heater units keep the surface temperatures constant. See Reference 26.

NUCLEAR-POWERED SHIPS

With the advent of the Savannah, which demonstrated feas-
ability of ship nuclear power, many other ships have been
built. Shielding is required for protection of personnel
and sensitive equipment.

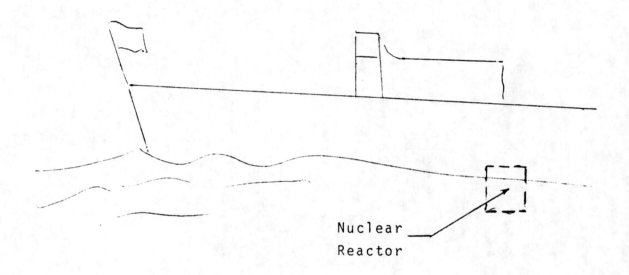

Nuclear
Reactor

Figure 4-3 A Nuclear-Powered Ship

The advantages are (a) reduction of air-borne atmospheric
pollution and (b) longer range.

NUCLEAR-POWERED AIRCRAFT CARRIER

Fig. 4-4

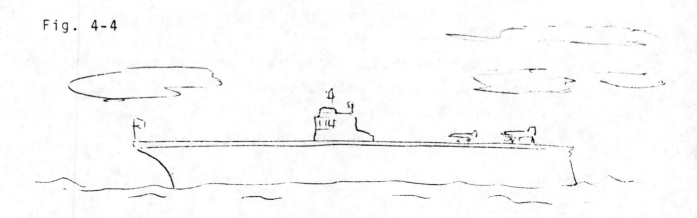

The United States was the first country to build a nuclear powered ship for its navy.

Specifics:

o It was built in 1965 and used in the Vietam Conflict in Southeast Asia.

o Capacity was almost 100 airplanes.

o It was powered by 8 nuclear reactors.

o Non-refueling range was increased, equivalent to 3 times around the world.

Advantages:

o The need for once/week refueling was eliminated.

o Speed and acceleration was increased.

o The power source was clean. Computers and other sensitive equipment was not contaminated with dirty oil particles.

NUCLEAR-POWERED SUBMARINES

With the advent of the first nuclear powered submarine, the
U.S.S. Nautalis, more submarines were built by U.S., Russia
and France over the years.

Reactor

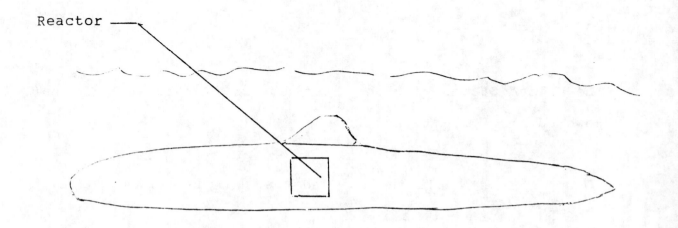

Figure 4-5   A Typical Nuclear Submarine

The advantage is their long range without the requirement
for frequent surfacing. Also, they are roomier than chemic-
ally-powered submarines. A typical military mission could
be as long as 180 days.

NUCLEAR REACTOR WASTES

At present, the radioactive wastes from nuclear machines, medical procedures and nuclear reactors are stored underneath the lands or oceans.

The United States wastes have been stored in concrete drums in the ocean or in large earth containers. Plans are in place for underground storage in New Mexico and other states (Ref. 22).

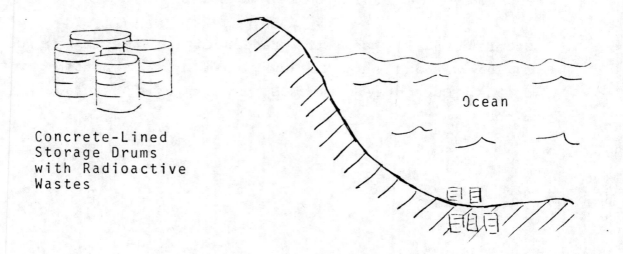

Concrete-Lined
Storage Drums
with Radioactive
Wastes

Ocean

A Disposal of Nuclear Wastes

Other countries, such as Japan, bury their wastes via an English company that contains them and buries them in the North Sea.

NUCLEAR WASTES (Cont.)

Regardless of all the hype concerning the disposal of nuclear wastes, it is really a non-problem. For three decades, disposal has been to contain the low-level wastes in steel drums and drop them in the bottom of the ocean. The drums are lined with 5 inches of concrete. Should small fissures occur in the containment and radioactivity leak out, the radiation levels are below natural background.

This method has been used since the early 1950's. Recently, sensitive visual and radiation detectors were lowered into the ocean to monitor the wastes. All containers were intact and no leaking radiation was measured.

Other countries seal the radioactive materials in ceramic cylinders and bury or drop them in the bottom of the oceans. Currently, the U.S. is exploring storage in deep mines.

Figure 4-7

Safe Nuclear Waste Disposal.

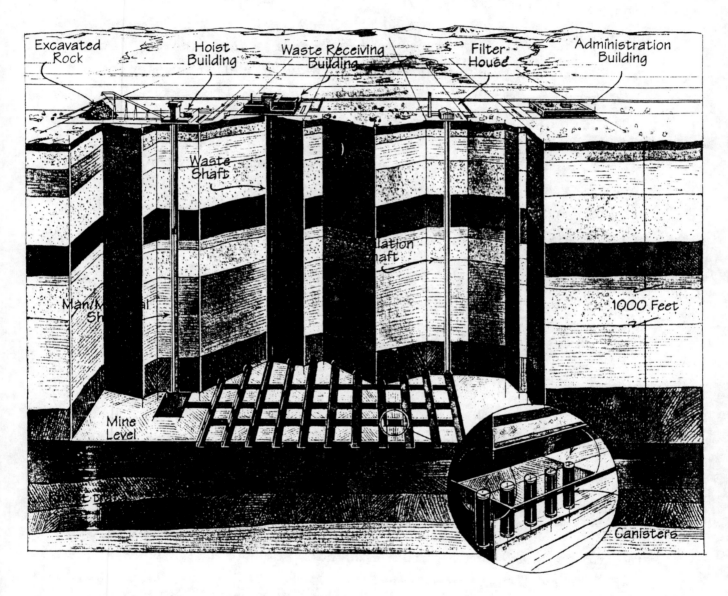

Underground rock formations have a long history of extreme stability and are monitored closely. Information courtesy U.S. Council for Energy Awareness, P.O. Box 66080, Dept. WA06, Washington, D.C. 20035.

NUCLEAR HAZARDS

History of Nuclear Hazards

The first recorded radioactive hazard encountered was in the late 1800's, when Roentgen placed a radiation source in his pocket and left it for several days. The skin on his thigh was reddened.

Through the years, there has been many small accidents with accelerators and nuclear reactors. Many were due to personnel error, such as thrusting a hand into the beam of a high energy accelerator when it was thought to be off.

In the bomb exposure of the natives of the Marshan Islands in the early 1950's, a wind change drove the radioactive particles in the wrong direction. Many suffered beta ray burns on their skin.

The first U.S. nuclear reactor accident occurred in the early 1950's, in Idaho. A lone operator of a small U.S. Army Research Reactor was lying on top of the reactor, and, for some reason, he pulled out the safety rod. The reactor went critical and he died. Nonetheless, that was the first nuclear reactor statistic.

Prior to that time. scientists had occasionally been killed or injured when experimenting with the amount of uranium necessary to obtain a critical mass.

The lesson here is that special safety procedures are necessary when dealing with nuclear energy.

NUCLEAR HAZARDS (Cont.)

The U.S. Three Mile Island Accident

One of the reactors at the Three Mile Island nuclear plant in Pennslyvania started to increase in power level in 1978. The visual and sound emitting alarms were activated.

The story, as told to the author, was that General Services Company, operator of the reactors had told the employees that, if they did something wrong during reactor operation, payment was to come out of their salaries. Consequently, none of the operators pushed the appropriate buttons to shut down the reaction. There were electronic control malfunctions also.

The Nuclear Regulatory Agency called reactor operators from Duke Power Company to the scene. Duke had operated 12 of the same type of reactors successfully for many years without a mishap. The out-of-town experts punched the correct buttons and stopped the reaction.

Fortunately, the local populace were exposed to low-levels of vented radioactivity and no one was injured.

The Russian Chernobyl Accident

In 1986, the Swedish ground radiation detectors recorded an increase in counting rate of airborne particles. After some detective work, it was determined that radioactive fallout was coming from the U.S.S.R.

Later, the Russian government admitted that they had experienced a reactor accident at Chernobyl and some personnel had died.

Many investigations of the cause of the reactor meltdown were held. It was determined that:
  a. The type of reactor involved was on inherently unstable reactor with positive reactivity. That is, as the temperature goes up, the core of the reactor becomes hotter. (All U.S. reactors are of negative stability).
  b. The reactor had no outer containment vessel as U.S. reactors do.
  c. The personnel were performing unauthorized experiments with the reactor including removing the safety rod from the core. These men were subsequently sentenced to prison.

U.S. doctors were sent to Moscow to attend the injured. The number of nearby civilians injured are reported to be in the tens of thousands.

Many animals died, including reindeer in other countries down wind to the fallout direction.

This is believed to be one of the worst if not the worst, radiation accident in history.

NUCLEAR HAZARDS (Cont.)

The Future of Nuclear Hazards

More attention will be given in the future to reducing the
nuclear hazards as more is known about them.

In Sweden, for example, it is planned to terminate the use
of nuclear reactors altogether. This is rather drastic.

Other scientists are making great strides in building safer
reactors (Ref. 33). Nuclear hazards are similar to commercial aircraft. They are quite safe if designed correctly
and operated within the design groundrules.

NUCLEAR ACCELERATORS

Large research accelerators exist that are used to study the collisions of high-speed particles.

    o Tevatron. This circular large accelerator is located at the Fermi National Accelerator Laboratory (Fermilab) at Batavia, Illinois.

New, even larger circular accelerators exist such as (CERN in Switzerland).

Larger accelerators are being built. For example, a Superconducting Supercollider (SSC) is being built in Texas, U.S.A. This machine can shoot two high-speed protons, each of energy 20 TeV together. This will be the most powerful machine yet and new physics concerning nuclear particles can be uncovered (Ref. 31).

Table 4-2 Some Types of High Energy Accelerators

There are many types of high speed accelerators, both linear (straight line) and cyclotron (circular). Some types are given below:

Type	No. In Operation
Linear	> 10
Cyclotron	> 56
Synchro-cyclotron	> 18
Proton synchrotron	> 6
Electron synchrotron	> 3
(Energy greater than 0.5 BeV)	
Betatron and low-energy	> 5
electron synchrotron	

NUCLEAR PARTICLE ACCELERATORS

Atomic and nuclear accelerators have been used for moving small particles to high velocities. The interactions with materials and biological tissues have been studied for over three decades (Ref. 11).

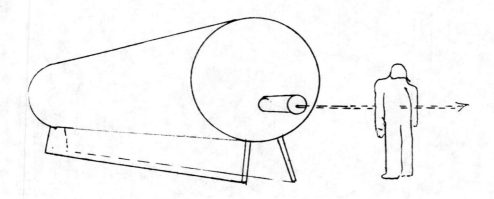

Figure 4-8

Sketch of a Research Accelerator

There are many applications, such as localized surface doping in electronic materials, killing cancerous cells and determination of physical scattering and stopping power of shielding. Typical energies are 1 MeV to 25 MeV. In general, the longer the accelerator tube, the higher the energy of the particles.

MEDICAL RADIATION MACHINES

Probably the most familiar radiation machine is the X-ray.
In this machine high speed electrons are produced that are
directed toward a copper target. Low energy electromagnetic
rays (X-rays) are produced by interactions with the electrons and the target metal. The result is X-rays whose
energy vary with the target material.

Fast electrons

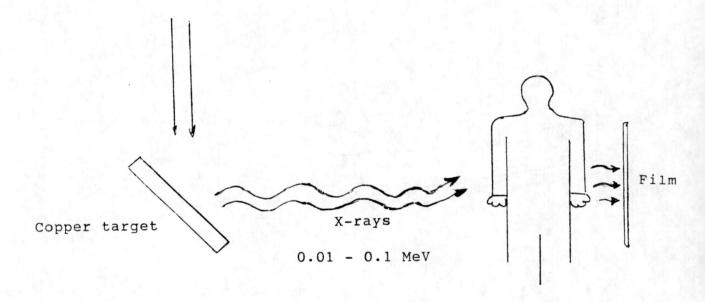

Copper target

X-rays

0.01 - 0.1 MeV

Film

Figure 4-9 Operation of an X-Ray Machine

A picture of internal organs are seen on a special X-ray
film due to the different biological densities.

MEDICAL MACHINES

Nuclear radiation from isotopes are used to scan the human
body to obtain an internal picture. Because the various
parts of the body have different densities that produce
scattering effects. Some of the machines are the following:

o Scanning Cobalt-60 Machines

o Nuclear Magnetic Resonance Machines

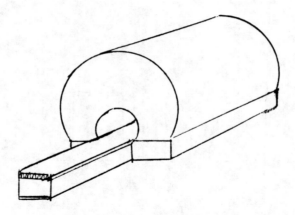

Figure 4-10   A Large Nuclear Magnetic Resonance Machine.
This Measures the Type and Location of Atoms
Within the Human Body.

NUCLEAR MEDICAL MACHINES (Cont.)

Cobalt Machines

As well as being used to scan the human body, collimated
radiation beams can kill cancerous cells. Either the
subject or the cobalt machine is rotated so that the
concentrated beam is on the irradiated cells.

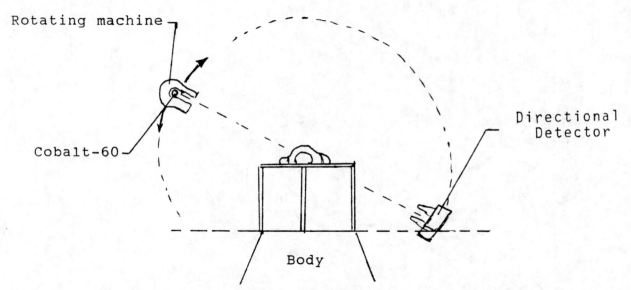

Figure 4-11 A Cobalt-60 Body Scanning Machine.

Cobalt-60 produces two high-energy gamma rays, 1.1 and 1.3
MeV. Because the radioactive cobalt is contained within a
thick lead container, the patient is not exposed until
container doors are opened.

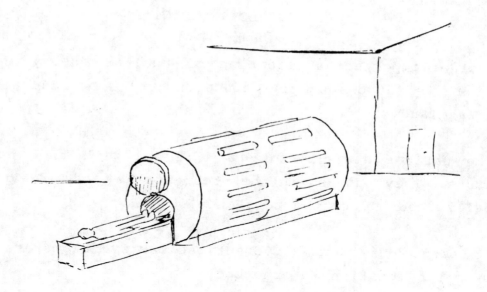

Figure 4-12 Sketch of a Whole Body Radiation Detector

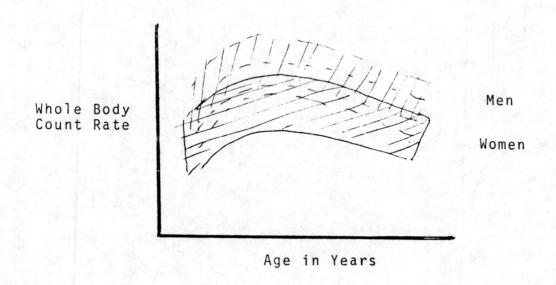

Whole Body
Count Rate

Men

Women

Age in Years

Figure 4-13 Calculated Internal Radioactivity(^{40}K) for Men and Women Based upon Measured Data.

NUCLEAR MEDICINE

Another important application of nuclear energy is the use of radioisotopes to kill cancerous cells or reduce activity of a gland.

The patient drinks or is injected with the radioactive atoms. They proceed in the blood stream and are preferenteally absorbed by the target cells.

It turns out that different radioactive atoms are used for specific locations of the body.

Besides killing the cells, the remaining radioisotopes decay, are exhaled or are excreted.

NUCLEAR WEAPONS PHENOMENA

Nuclear weapons are becoming more and more a part of our daily lives. The race for the development of an atomic bomb was initiated in October 1940 by Hirohito in Japan. See Ref. 28 for details.

Other countries joined the race in the 1940's and 1950's. The United States was the first to drop atomic bombs in World Was II. Approximately 76,000 people were killed at Hiroshima on August 3, 1945 and 38,000 at the submarine base (Nagasaki) on August 6, 1945. Little was known of the effects of nuclear weapons in those days. The pilots of the planes were lucky to have survived due to the intense heat and radiations.

Over the last three decades, major world powers have performed weapons testing to; (a) determine prompt effects and (b) improve the efficiency of the explosives and (c) determine fallout effects.

There is a wide variety of effects from the nuclear weapons depending upon the medium. Examples of four environments are given below.

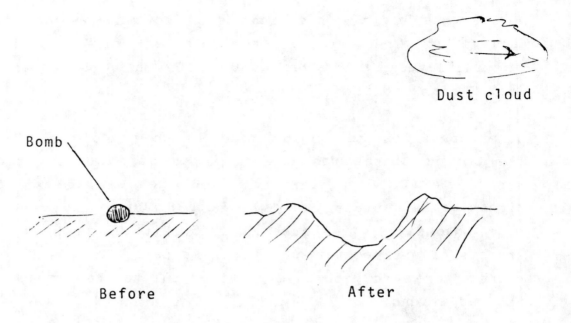

Figure 4-14 A Nuclear Burst at Ground Level

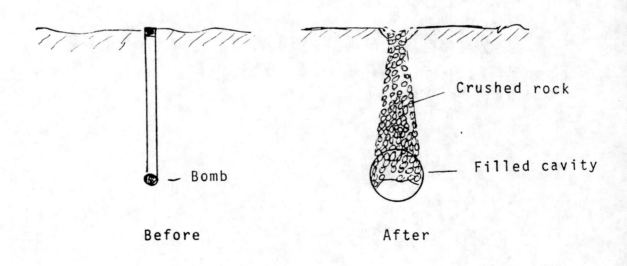

Figure 4-15 An Underground Nuclear Explosion

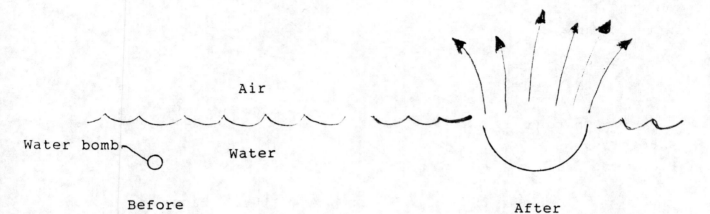

Air

Water bomb

Water

Before

After

Figure 4-16
An Underwater Explosion

Dirt and dust become airborne

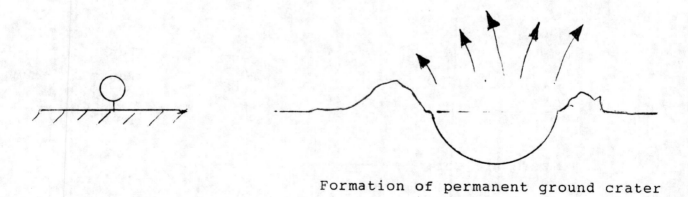

Formation of permanent ground crater

Figure 4-17
A Ground Explosion

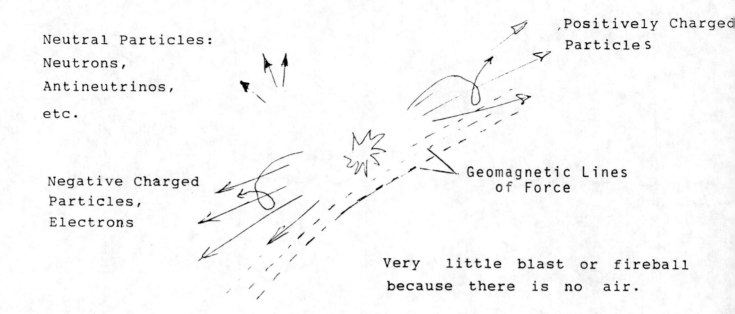

Neutral Particles:
Neutrons,
Antineutrinos,
etc.

Positively Charged Particles

Negative Charged
Particles,
Electrons

Geomagnetic Lines of Force

Very little blast or fireball because there is no air.

Figure 4-18 A Typical Nuclear Weapon Burst in Space

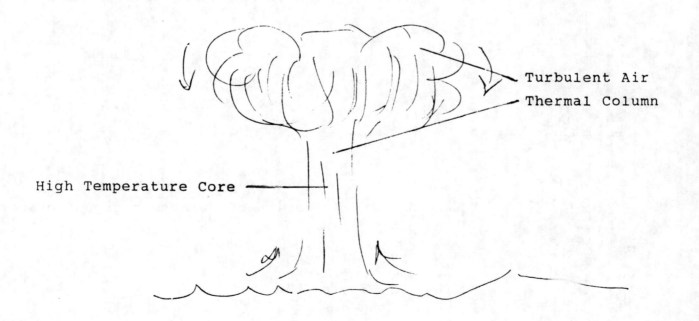

Turbulent Air
Thermal Column

High Temperature Core

Figure 4-19 A Nuclear Weapon Burst in the Atmosphere

Table

Who Has Nuclear Weapons?

Countries That Have
Declared They Have
Nuclear Bombs

    China

    Commonwealth of

    Independent States

    France

    United Kingdom

    United States

Countries Strongly
Suspected of Having
Nuclear Bombs

    India

    Israel

    Pakistan

Countries Working On
Nuclear Bombs

    Algeria

    Iran

    Iraq

    Libya

    North Korea

Countries Suspected of
Having Nuclear Bombs

    Argentina

    Brazil

    South Africa

Source: USA Today, p. 13A, January 1992.

4-29

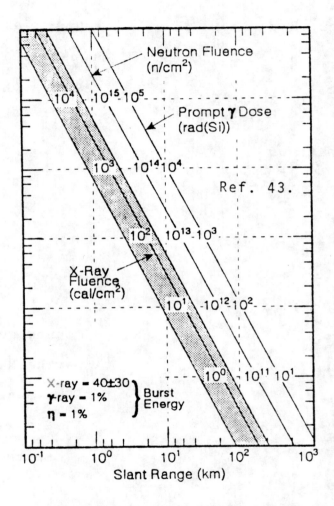

X-ray fluence, neutron fluence and prompt γ-ray dose as a function of separation for a 1 MT exo-atmospheric burst with x-rays = 40±30%, γ-ray = 1% and n = 1% of the burst energy.

Figure 4-20

ANIMAL BIOLOGICAL RESPONSES

During the U.S. weapons tests in the Pacific, rabbits, mice and other animals were exposed to neutrons, gamma rays and X-rays at various distances from the explosion.

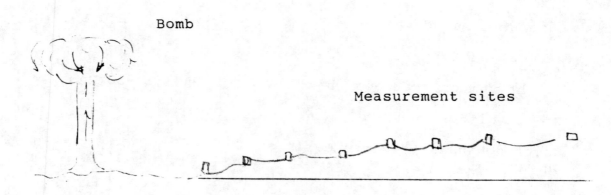

Bomb

Measurement sites

Figure 4-21

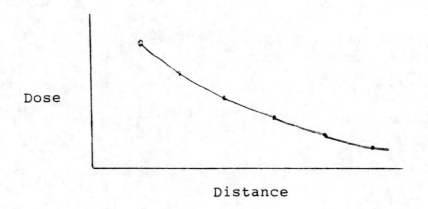

Dose

Distance

In this way the responses of animals to various forms of nuclear radiation were investigated.

The extrapolation of the biological responses to humans gave important information (Ref. 29).

Table 4-4

The Biological Effects of <u>Brief</u> Radiation Exposure

Biological Radiation Effect	Single Exposure
Sure and sudden death	5000 Rem
50% chance of surviving	450 Rem
99% chance of surviving	250 Rem
Cataracts may develop	200 Rem
Nausea and fatigue	100 Rem
Slight temporary blood changes	50 Rem
Growth disturbance to human fetus	37 ± 13 Rem
Subtle changes to nerve cells of unborn rats	15 ± 5 Rem
Maximum yearly legal dose	5 Rem
May double likelihood of childhood leukemia	1 Rem
The average annual dose for 1,250,000 radiation workers in 1975	0.34 Rem
Typical chest x-ray	0.3 Rem
The average dose per year in the U.S. from natural sources (terrestrial and cosmic)	0.2 ± 0.1 Rem

o Reference 43, page 11.

RADIATION EFFECTS ON BIOLOGICAL SYSTEMS

The effects of penetrating nuclear radiation on biological systems, such as rabbits or individual cells is much more complicated than solid or liquid inanimate materials.

The primary reasons are that:

- o Radiation effects vary with the species.
- o The response varies with many factors--
  - Direction of the radiation.
  - Self-shielding of internal organs.
  - Penetration characteristics of the radiation beam.
  - Type of exposure, such as breathing, drinking or external exposure.
- o Biological systems can undergo repair and erase the radiation damage.

For further details, see Ref. 29.

Table 4-5

Decrease in Human Life Span with
Various Risk Factors*

Source of Risk	Average Life Span Reduction -days	Probability of Cancer -percent
Nonradiation		
Home accidents	95	-----
Moderate drinking	150	-----
Automobile accidents	200	-----
Farming	277	-----
Mining	328	-----
20% overweight	985	-----
Smoking (one pack/day)	2370	-----
Radiation		
1 rem	1	25.03
1 rem/year for 30 years	30	26
5 rem/year for 30 years	150	29
10 rem	10	25.3
100 rem	~ 100	28.0
Medical X-rays	6	-----
Natural background radiation	8	

* Source
Passenheim, Burr C., How To Do Radiation Tests, Ingenuity
Inc., San Diego, California 92117, 1988, P. 13.

RADIOACTIVE CARBON DATING

The age of former living material, such as trees, may be determined by counting the amount of carbon present. It works because all living systems have small amounts of radioactive carbon. The carbon atom emits radiation that can be measured and its decay observed.

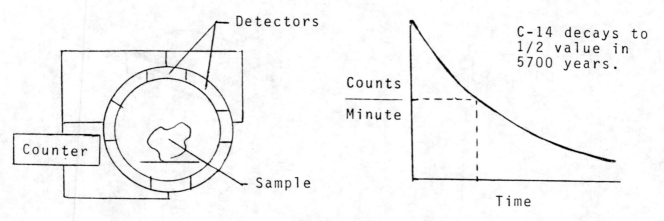

Figure 4-22

By the use of radioactive decay half-life charts, the age of the specimen can be determined.

The decay of other elements can be measured to verify the age.

NUCLEAR BATTERIES

Long-lived nuclear batteries have been researched for the last three decades. They have their advantages and disadvantages.

Recently, new types of radioactive batteries have been developed and should be available commercially.

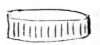
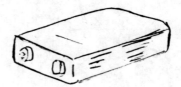

Advantages are the following:
    o Long-life.
    o Near-constant power

Various types of batteries are possible due to the wide variety of radioactive materials available.

FOOD IRRADIATION

-Sterilization and life-extension

There are many advantages to the irradiation of meat, fruits
and vegetables with cobalt-60 gamma rays.

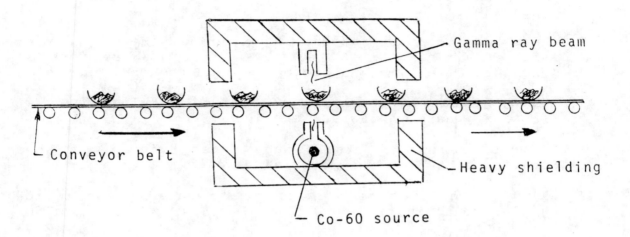

Figure 4-23   The Process of Food Irradiation

Specifics are:

o Food research tests have been performed since 1963 on
the various types of meats, poultry, fruits and vegetables. Reactor tests produce worse by-products so
gamma rays are recommended.

o Cobalt-60 radiation is the safest."Radioactive fears
are groundless," said Dr. Joel Gray, a medical physicist at the Mayo Clinic. "Radiation is not   left in
the food."

o Cooking changes the food more than radiation.

o Food spoilage is delayed and disease-causing bacteria
are virtually eliminated.

o One irradition facility in Mulberry, Florida is operated by Vindication of Florida, Inc.

Table 4-6

Rules for Handling or Working
Near Radioactivity*

1. Keep radioactive and non radioactive work areas separated.

2. Keep the amount of radioactive material you are working with at a minimum. If there are many parts, work on one part at a time and store the rest behind a shield.

3. Always wear appropriate protective clothing (gloves, lab coat, safety glasses, etc.).

4. Always monitor yourself and wash your hands when leaving a radioactive materials area.

5. Always monitor the working area regularly for radioactive contamination.

6. Always label all radioactive items clearly, indicating isotope, total activity, physical form and date.

7. Never eat, drink or smoke in or near a radioactive materials area.

8. Never allow personal items to come in contact with radioactive material.

9. Never work with unprotected cuts or breaks in the skin, particularly on the hands or forearms.

10. Dispose of radioactive materials only in authorized and marked containers.

11. Always use tongs or remote handling equipment when handling radioactive material to reduce dose.

12. Always report real or suspected contamination to health physics.

13. Never attempt to perform decontamination without assistance from health physics.

* Reference 43.

SUMMARY

In this chapter, I have attempted to give an overview of the many faces of nuclear energy as it affects everyone.

Nuclear energy is being used in many applications, from new long-lived landing field lights to unique space propulsion devices. The applications are too extensive to be included herein. However, a few of the more important aspects are treated.

Although nuclear energy can be very beneficial to mankind, it must be handled correctly. There is no room for carelessness or poor management of nuclear systems.

Everyone experiences radiation every day. Indeed, the cosmic rays penetrate down into the deepest mines. Fortunately, they are of low intensities. This is not true as mankind travels beyond the earth's atmosphere.

Some aspects of extra-terrestrial travel are treated in the following section.

Chapter 5

SPACE RADIATION

In the preceding chapters, we have seen that there are a wide variety of nuclear particles that cause many effects in both materials and biological systems.

When man leaves the Earth and travels beyond the safety of our atmosphere, he can be expected to suffer deleterious effects unless shielded from the penetrating radiations from the solar cosmic rays, galactic cosmic rays and the radiations from nuclear power systems. The radiation belts of the planets being visited can be an important radition source also.

Because of the tremendous distances to the stars and the fact that no adequate propulsion systems exists, we will not be able to travel beyond our solar system.

Because we are at the mercy of the gigantic solar part-icle eruptions from our sun, our space travel must be carried on as fast as possible to avoid both system and biological damage. Consequently, extremely powerful nucl-ear propulsion units are needed. The slow, chemical propulsion systems are just the model Ts of the space travel.

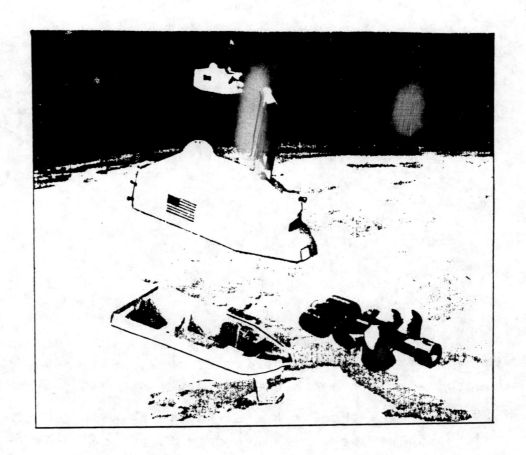

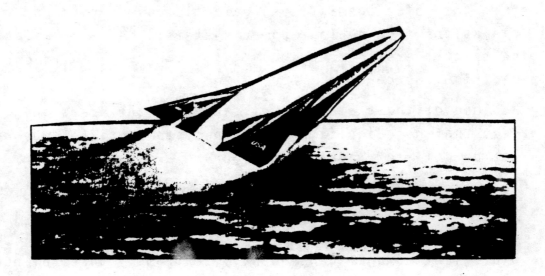

RADIATION IN SPACE TRAVEL

High energy nuclear particles can be encountered in space travel. Most, if not all near-earth satellites are under the protection of the magnetic field of the earth which reaches far out into space (Ref 32). This reduces the galactic and solar cosmic rays by bending them away from near-earth space.

During the Apollo spacecraft that visited the moon in the early 1970's, the astronauts were exposed to direct radiation from the sun and galaxies.

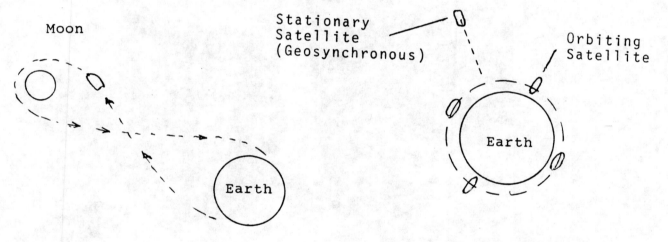

Apollo Mission

Satellites

Figure 5-1 Apollo and Satellites

Fortunately, only one major solar flare occurred. The astronauts were estimated to have received a 1 rem dose (a negligible amount).

Astronauts on extended space travel must deal with radiation from planetary radiation belts and nuclear pro-pulsion units.

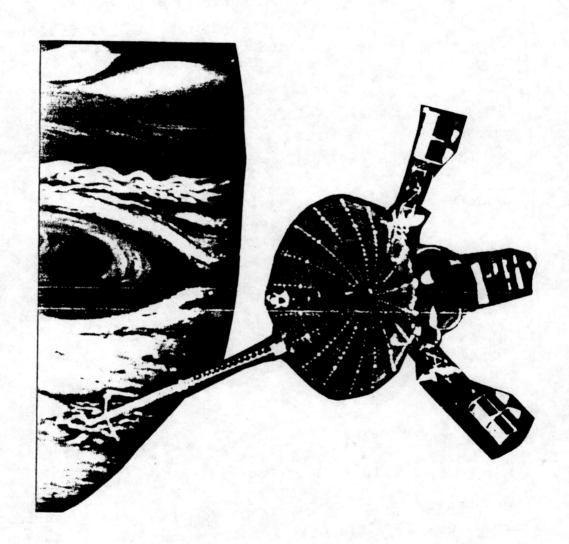

Near-Earth Space

As one travels higher and higher in the atmosphere, increased amounts of solar and cosmic radiation are encountered.

Definitive radiation studies at high altitudes for conditions during intense particle bombardment from the Sun have yet to be undertaken.

However, when one leaves the entire protection of the Earth's atmosphere, definite increased numbers of nuclear particles are expected to be intercepted. See Figures 5-1-5-3.

Extended Space Travel

If man is going to travel far from the Earth, it appears that the planet Mars is the most friendly. Water has recently been discovered on it and it is not too far away. See Figure 5-4.

Radition will be received by the space travelers from a number of sources, such as:

o Geomagnetically trapped particles
o Solar cosmic rays
o Galactic cosmic rays
o Nuclear propulsion units

The three areas of concern are electronics, materials and biological radiation damage.

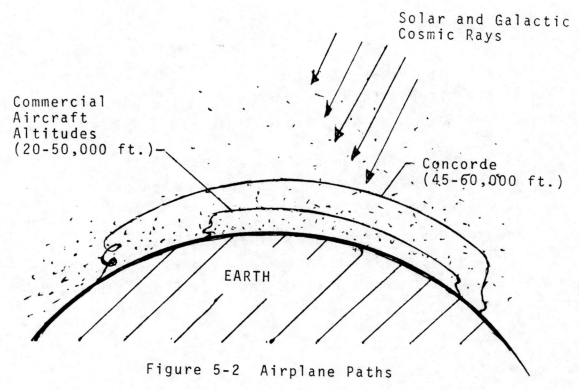

Solar and Galactic
Cosmic Rays

Commercial
Aircraft
Altitudes
(20-50,000 ft.)

Concorde
(45-60,000 ft.)

EARTH

Figure 5-2 Airplane Paths

- Not to Scale

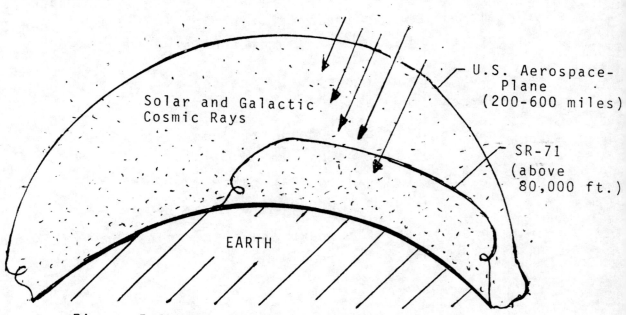

U.S. Aerospace-
Plane
(200-600 miles)

SR-71
(above
80,000 ft.)

Solar and Galactic
Cosmic Rays

EARTH

Figure 5-3 High Altitude Airplane Paths

MANNED SPACE TRAVEL
- Probably the First Manned Space Travel Mission

Transit Time Each Way: Nuclear Propulsion- 0.9 Months

Chemical Propulsion: 9 Months

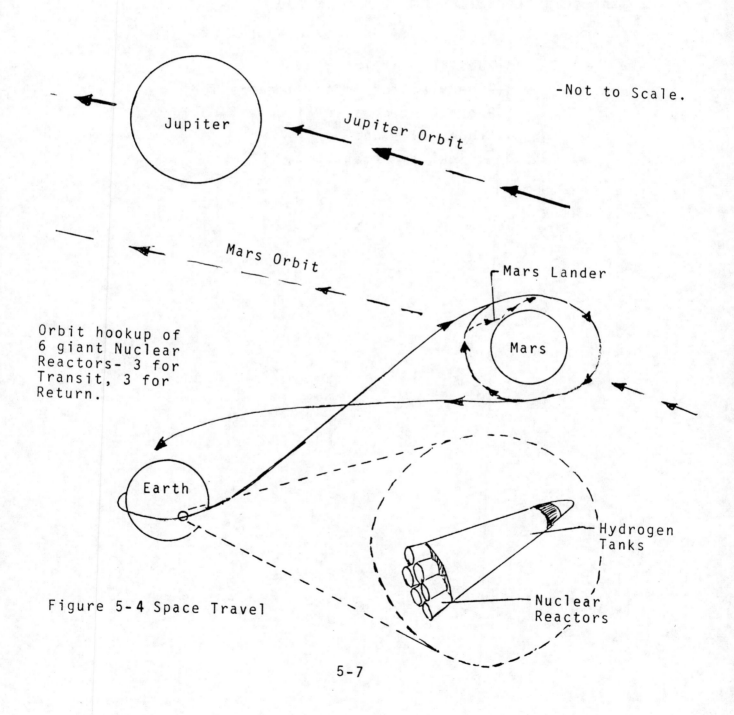

Figure 5-4 Space Travel

Biological Radiation Damage.

Assumming the travels are carried on when the sun is inactive, the solar radiation can be minimized.

Biological damage can be minimized by the use of:

- o Radition shielding
- o Prophylactics before irradiation
- o Prophylactics after irradiation
- o Proper diet and
- o Medical treatment.

BIOLOGICAL RECOVERY FROM RADIATION
EXPOSURE DURING SPACE TRAVEL(Ref. 25).

o Astronauts survive the
  Galactic and Solar Cosmic
  Rays by Healthy Regime.

o Recovery Curves Were Defined
  by Dr. Blair in the 1950s.

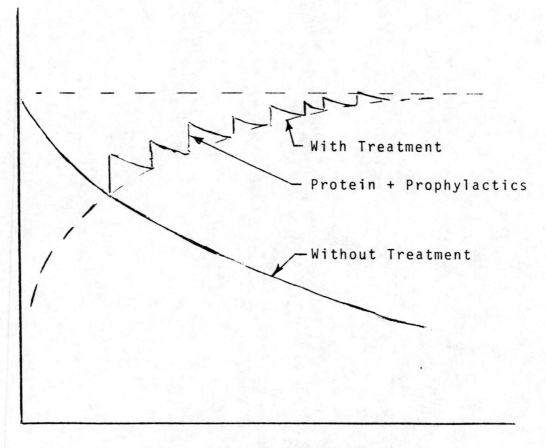

Figure 5-5   Radiation Protection during Space Flight.

Chapter 6

FUTURE OF NUCLEAR ENERGY

Although it has been almost a hundred years since radio-activity was discovered, there is much yet to be learned. Many of the radioactive decay schemes must be determined more precisely. The effects of terrestrial and space radiation on plants, animals, humans and materials are yet to be explored.

We live in an exciting age. Vast new advances are expected from the development of new, more powerful medical and scientific machines.

New materials are being developed that are more radiation resistance for terrestrial and space uses. New types of reactors are on the drawing boards, such as fission-fusion reactors and gaseous space nuclear propulsion devices. Research is proceeding on the plasma fusion reactor and cold fusion.

The future appears bright indeed!

REFERENCES

1. Taylor, P.D. and Larwood, G.P., eds., Major Evolutionary Radiations, Clarendon(Oxford Univ. Pr.) New York, NY 1990.

2. Wagner, Henry N., Living with Radiation, The Risk, The Promise, John Hopkins Univ. Press, 1989.

3. Ziegler, J.F., Handbook of Stopping Cross-Sections for Energetic Ions in All Elements, Pergamon Press, New York,, NY 1980.

4. Knoll, G.G., Radiation Detection and Measurement, John Wiley and Sons, Inc., New York, NY 1979.

5. Stassinopoulos, E. G., Radiation Environments of Space, IEEE Short Course, Reno, NV July 1990.

6. Brown, Dennis B., Total Dose Effects at Dose Rates Typical of Space, ibid.

7. Buehler, M.G., and Blaes, B.R., Alpha - Particle Sensi--tive Test SRAMS, IEEE Trans. Nucl. Science, Vol. 37, No. 6, p. 1852, December 1990.

8. Dyer, Dr. C.S., et al, Measurements of Solar Flare Environments... , Trans. Nucl. Sci., Vo Vol. 37, 6 No. 6, pp. 1929-1937, December 1990.

9. Johnston, A.H. and Hughlock, B.W., Latchup in CMOS from Single Particles, IEEE Trans.Nucl. Sci., Vol. 37, No. 6, December 1990.

10. McMorrow, Dale, Knudson, Alvin R. and Campbell, Arthur B., Fast Charge Collection ..., IEEE Trans. Nucl. Sci. , Vol. 37, No. 6, pp. 1902-1908, December 1990.

REFERENCES (Cont.)

11. Wilson, Robert R. and Littauer, Raphael, Accelerators, Machines of Nuclear Physics, Anchor Books, Doubleday & Company, Inc., Garden City, New York, 1960.

12. Glasstone, Samuel, Ed., The Effects of Nuclear Weapons, Superintendent of Documents, U.S. Government Printing Office, Washington, D.C., 1962.

13. Bouquet, F. L., Radiation Damage in Materials, 3rd Ed., Systems Co., P.O. Box 876, Graham, WA, 98338, 1990.

14. Bouquet, F.L., Radiation Effects on Electronics, 3rd Ed., Systems Company, 1990.

15. Bouquet, F.L., Radiation Effects on Kapton, 1st Edition, Systems Company, 1990.

16. Bouquet, F.L., Radiation Effects on Teflon, Volumes 1 and 2, 1st Edition, Systems Company, 1989.

17. Wilson, R. R., "Particle Accelerations," Scientific American, March 1958.

18. Livingston, M. S., High Energy Accelerators, Inter-science Publishers, New York, NY 1954.

19. Claus, W. D., Ed., Radiation Biology and Medicine, Addison-Wesley Publishing Co., Reading, MA 1958.

20. Freeman, Ray, A Handbook of Nuclear Magnetic Resonance, University of Cambridge, United Kingdom, 1987.

21. Bouquet, F. L., Solar Energy Simplified, 4th Edition, Systems Company, 1991.

REFERENCES (Cont.)

22. Anon, Quake Shakes Nuclear-Waste Space, Science News, Volume 141, January 18, 1992.

23. Lemonick, Michael D., The Ultimate Quest, Time, p. 50-56, April 16, 1990.

24. Morgan, K. Z. and Turner, J. E., Principles of Radiation Protection, John Wiley & Sons, Inc., New York NY, 1967.

25. Bouquet, F. L., Introduction to Biological Radiation Effects, Systems Company, 1992.

26. Bouquet, F. L., Spacecraft Design-Thermal and Radiation Systems Company, 1991.

27. Glasstone, Samuel, Sourcebook on the Space Sciences, D. Van Nostrand Company, Inc., New York, NY 1965.

28. Manning, Paul, Hirohito-The War Years, Bantum Books, 666 Fifth Avenue, New York, NY 10103, 1989.

29. Bouquet, F. L. Introduction to Biological Radiation Effects, Systems Company, 1992.

30. Ray, Dixy Lee and Guzzo, Lou, Trashing the Planet, Regnery Gateway Publishing Co., Washington, D.C., 1990.

31. Jackson, J. David, et al, The Superconducting Super-collider, Sci. Am., Vol. 254, No. 3, pp. 66-77, March 1986.

32. Hones, Edward W., Jr., The Earth's Magnetotail, Sci. Am., pp. 40-47, March 1986.

33. Lester, Richard K., Rethinking Nuclear Power, Sci. Am., Vol. 254, No. 3, pp. 31-39, March 1986.

34. Taylor, Theodore B., Third-Generation Nuclear Weapons, Sci. Am., Vol. 256, No. 4., pp. 30-39, April 1930.

35. Anon, Who Has Nuclear Weapons, USA Today, p. 13A, January 9, 1992.

36. Heyde, Kris, The Nuclear Shell Model, Springer-Verlag, New York, NY 1989.

37. Anon., McGraw-Hill Encyclopedia of Science and Technology, Vol. 7, p. 691, 1977.

38. Schwarschild, B., Four of Five New Experiments Claim Evidend for the 17 keV Neurtrino, Physics Today, pp. 17-19, May 1991.

39. Close, Frank et al, The Particle Explosion, Oxford Press, 1987.

40. Winter, Klaus (Ed.), Neutrino Physics, Cambridge University Press, 40 West 20th Street, New York, NY ($125) 1991.

41. Jagger, John, The Nuclear Lion, What Every Citizen Should Know About Nuclear Power and Nuclear War, Plenum New York, NY.

42. Casten, Richard F., Nuclear Structure from a Simple Perspective, Oxford Press, New York, NY, (376 pages, $59) 1990.

REFERENCES (Cont.)

43. Passenheim, Burr C., How To Do Radiation Tests, Ingenuity Ink, 5538 Camber Drive, San Diego, California 92117 -5838.

45. Taubes, Gary, A Cold Fusion Deja Vu at Caltech, Science, Vol. 254, No. 5038, p. 1582, December 13, 1991

46. Conn, Robert W., The International Thermonuclear Experimental Reactor, Sci. Am., Vol. 266, No. 4, pp. 102-110 April 1992.

BIBLIOGRAPHY

Alpen, Edward L., Radiation Biophysics, Prentice-Hall, Englewood Cliffs, NJ, 1990.

Anon., McGraw-Hill Encyclopedia of Science and Technology, Vol. 7, p. 691, 1977.

Anon., The Solar System: A Practical Guide, Allen and Unwin Publ., North Sidney, Australia (225 pages, $19.95), (Distributed by Paul and Co., Concord, MA in the United States)

Anon., Who Has Nuclear Weapons, USA Today, p. 13A, January 9, 1992.

Berger, Melvin, Atoms, Molecules and Quarks, Putnam Publ., 1986.

Berger, Melvin, Our Atomic World, Watts Publ., 1989.
Betss, R. R. and Kolata, J. J., Eds., Nuclear Structure and Heavy Ion Reaction Dynamics, Inst. of Physics, Philadelphia PA, 1990.

Bronowski, J. and Selsam, M. E., Biography of an Atom, Harper Publ. Co., 1987.

Cahn, R. N. and Goldhaber, G., The Experimental Foundations of Particle Physics, Cambridge University Press, ($28.00) 1990.

Casten, Richard F., Nuclear Structure from a Simple Perspective, Oxford University Press, New York, NY, 1990.

Close, Frank et al, The Particle Explosion, Oxford Press, 1987.

BIBLIOGRAPHY (Cont.)

Conn, Robert W., The International Thermonuclear Experimental Reactor, Sci. Am., Vol. 266, No. 4, pp. 102-110, April 1992.

Dawson, John M., Plasma Particle Accelerators, Sci. Am., p. 54, March 1989.

Gavin, Richard L., (Cold) Fusion: The Evidence Reviewed, Science, p. 1394, November 29, 1991.

Gillespies, Charles Coulston (Ed.), Dictionary of Scientific Biography, Vol. 1, Charles Schribner and Sons, New York, NY, 1970.

Gordey, J. Geoffrey et al, Progress toward a Tokamak Fusion Reactor, Physics Today, Vol. 45, No. 1, pp. 22-30, January 1992.

Heyde, Kris, The Nuclear Shell Model, Springer-Verlag, New York, NY, 1989.

Hill, T. W. and Dessler, A. J., Plasma Motions in Planetary Magnetospheres, Science, Vol. 252, pp. 410-415, April 19, 1991.

Jagger, John, The Nuclear Lion, What Every Citizen Should Know About Nuclear Power and Nuclear War, Plenum, New York, NY, (402 pages), 1991.

Mann, W. B., Rytz, A. and Spernol, A., Radioactivity Measurements, Principles and Practice, Pergamon Press, Oxford, UK, (202 pages, $40), 1992.

Neil, Ardley, The World of the Atom, Glouchester Press, 1989.

Parker, Barry, Search For a Supertheory From Atoms to Superstrings, Plenum Press, 1987.

Passenheim, Burr C., How To Do Radiation Tests, Ingenuity Ink, 5838 Camber Drive, San Diego, California 5838-92117.

Schwarschild, B., Four of Five New Experiments Claim Evidend for the 17 keV Neutrino, Physics Today, pp. 17-19, May 1991.

Schwartz, John H., Elementary Particles and The Universe. Essays in Honor of Murray Gell-Mann, Cambridge University Press, New York, NY (212 pages, $49.95), 1991.

Smith, Henrick, Intro to Quantum Mechanics, World Scientific, Teaneck, NJ, (285 pages, $58), 1991.

Sykes, Lynn R. and Davis, Dan M., The Yields of Soviet Strategic Weapons, Sci. Am., Vol. 256, No. 1, pp. 29-37, January 1987.

Taubes, Gary, A Cold Fusion Deja Vu at Caltech, Science, Vol. 254, No. 5038, p. 1582, December 13, 1991.

Tipler, Paul A., Physics for Scientists and Engineers, 3rd Edition, Worth Publishers, New York, NY (1426 pages, $64.95), 1991.

Trower, W. Peter, Lonely Hearts of the Cosmos: The Scientific Quest for Secret Universe, Harper Collins Publ., New York, NY, (438 pages, $25), 1991.

Williams, W. S. C., Nuclear and Particle Physics, Clarendon (Oxford University Press), New York, NY (385 pages), 1991.

BIBLIOGRAPHY (Cont.)

Winter, Klaus (Ed.), Neutrino Physics, Cambridge University
Press, 40 West 20th Street, New York, NY ($125) 1991.

GLOSSARY

absorbed dose

The absorbed dose, D, is the mean energy imparted to the material by the incident ionizing radiation. It is dependent on the magnitude of the radiation field and on the degree of interaction between the radiation and the material. The SI name for the unit of absorbed dose is the Gray (GY).

$$1 \text{ GY} = \text{J kg}^{-1}$$

The special unit of absorbed dose, rad, may be used temporarily.

$$1 \text{ rad} = 10^{-2} \text{ J kg}^{-1}$$

absorbed dose rate

The absorbed dose rate, D, is increment of absorbed dose in a given time interval.

$$\dot{D} = \frac{dD}{dt}$$

The SI unit is $\text{J kg}^{-1} \text{ s}^{-1}$. The special unit, rad s^{-1}, may be used temporarily.

alpha particle	A massive positively charged particle (He^{++}) emitted by cerain radioactive materials; particle energy depends on the partain material penetrating ability is limited.
Atom	Each element is made up of a specific electron and nuclear configuration. An element may be composed of one to seven other atoms. For example, natural uranium consists of uranium 238(99.3%) and uranium 235(0.714%).
Atomic Bomb	A fission or fusion device that is capable of driving a nuclear reaction.
Aurora Borealis	Spectacular colored light effects that occur near the artic and antartic regions. Although a mystery for many years, it is now known to be caused by nuclear particles trapped in the tail of the Earth's magnetosphere.
Alamogordo	Alamogordo, New Mexico was the site of the first U.S. nuclear (fission) explosion on July 16, 1945. It had a yield of 17 kilotons of TNT.

Atomic particles

Atom refers to the characteristics of an entire atom composed of an electron shell around a nucleus. When the atom is moving fast enough, such as in the sun, it is stripped of the outer electrons and is essentially a nuclear particle. Hence, the words atomic and nuclear are used interchangeably sometimes in this book.

beta

A particle emitted by certain radioactive materials. A negatively charged beta has the characteristics of an electron; a positively charged beta particle is a positron.

bremsstrahlung

Electromagnetic radiation (photon) emitted when energetic charged particles lose energy to the influence of the electric field of absorber atoms.

(C)

Carbon as in rads (C).

crosslink

Chemical bond formed between separate polymer elements; crosslinking may be intermolecular (between molecules) or intramolecular (between parts of the same molecule).

Characteristic X-rays   Each atom, when stimulated, will
                          release X-rays that are specific
                          to that atom.

Computer Tomography   This refers to a process whereby
                          the human body can be mapped using
                          a radiation source and radiation
                          detectors. Sophisticated computer
                          electronics evaluates the detector
                          results and presents the data into
                          useful form.

Critical (operation)   A nuclear reactor is said to be
                          critical when the control rods are
                          slid out of the core. The core
                          then begins to generate heat
                          because it now has a critical mass
                          (minimum amount of fissionable
                          material to sustain a nuclear
                          reaction).

depth dose   The absorbed radiation dose at a
                              particular depth in a specific
                              absorber; depth-dose curves show
                              the distribution of   absorbed
                              energy in a material.

displacement   Physical relocation of nuclei of
                              an absorber through collision
                              process, resulting in disruption
                              of the materials crystal struct-
                              ure.

dose   The absorbed dose (D) is the
                              quotient of ΔE_D by Δm, where ΔE_D
                              is the energy imparted by ionizing
                              radiation to the matter in a
                              volume element and Δm, is the
                              mass of matter in that volume
                              element

$$D = \frac{\Delta E_D}{\Delta m} \text{ in ergs per gram}$$
$$1 \text{ rad} = 100 \text{ ergs/gram.}$$

dose rate effects   An effect on a material which is
                              different in magnitude or type
                              (for the same total dose), de-
                              pending on the irradiation rate.

electron (beta particle)   A charged particle carrying a
                              unit electronic charge either
                              positive (positron) or negative

(negatron). The term electron is commonly used instead of negatron when discussing the negatively charged particle. The mass of an electron is 1/1835 of the mass of a proton.

electron volt   A measure of energy of a charged particle, about 1.6×10^{-5} watt-seconds. (one ft-lb. equals approx. 0.85×10^{10} Bev.).

eV   Electron volt.

excitation   A process by which energy is supplied to electrons, atoms, or radicals, rendering them chemically more reactive.

exposure   The exposure dose is a measure of the radiation based upon its ability to produce ionization. Exposure dose is expressed in Roentgens of x or gamma radiation.

fluence   The product of the flux (particle density x velocity), and time, which indicates the total number of particles that have passed through a unit area, usually one cm^2.

flux   Number of particles passing through unit area per unit time.

free radical

An atom or radical group of atoms having one electron not involved in bond formation; free radicals are highly reactive and may be highly mobile.

gamma ray

Highly penetrating electromagnetic radiation from the nuclei of radioactive substances. They are of the same nature as x-rays differing only in their origin.

Hadron

Small nuclear particle

Hardened

The process of making material or component less sensitive to the effects of penetrating radiation. Typical methods are the following:

- o Placing thin shielding material around the component as an absorber.
- o Use shielding to scatter the radiation.
- o Use multiple layers of shielding to degrade the radiation.
- o Adding radiation absorbing chemicals, such as anti-rads.
- o Circumvention. Redesign of electronic circuits to be insensitive to radiation.

Hazards	Radioactive hazards, such as escaping radiation from sources or nuclear reactors, may occur if the radiation is not controlled. Over the last 40 years, radiation hazards from the uncontrolled release of radioactivity have been miniscule. No one died from the 3-Mile Island Event. Ill-designed plants, such as Chernobyl (no containment) caused many human and animal deaths.
Implosion	Implosion is a term used to describe a type of nuclear bomb that components are driven together to form a critical mass. This is in counter-distinction to gun-type bombs where fractional fission masses are fired toward each other.
ion	An electrically charged atom, radical, or molecule resulting from the addition or removal of electrons by any number of possible processes.
ionization	The process of ion formation.
irradiation	Exposure to radiation.

keV   One thousand electron volts.

Kiloton   The primary term used to describe
                            the energy yield of a nuclear
                            explosion. It refers to the amount
                            of energy emitted by a similar ex-
                            plosion of TNT (trinitrotoluene).
                            Other terms used are Megaton (for
                            large bombs, 10^6 tons) and
                            sub-kiloton for small bombs.

Lepton   Small nuclear particle

LET   Linear Energy Transfer - the ra-
                            diation energy lost per unit
                            length of path through a mater-
                            ial, usually expressed in kilo-
                            electron volts per micron of
                            path; a higher LET value indic-
                            ates more effective ionization
                            of the absorber.

Linac   This term is short for linear
                            accelerator. The largest U.S.
                            linac is 20 BeV. It is 3 miles
                            long and located in Palo Alto,
                            California.

Mass	The amount of atoms contained in a material. It is composed primarily of electrons, protons and neutrons and secondarily of various other particles.
Nagaski	Nagaski, Japan was where the second bomb was dropped in World War II. It occurred on August 9, 1945 and its yield was 17 kilotons.
neutron	An uncharged elementary particle present in the nucleus of every atom heavier than hydrogen. Neutrons are released during fission. Their mass is approximately equal to that of a proton.
neutron activation	A process by which absorber atoms become radioactive through capture of a neutron by the nucleus of the absorber.
Nuclear	The word "nuclear" refers to the mass composing the atom. It is composed of neutrons and protons.
PET	Positive Electron Tomography. A medical process that makes use of radioactive atoms that produce positrons.

photon	An electromagnetic quantity. Its energy is proportional to the frequency of the associated wave.
Positron	A positively charged electron emitted by natural radioactive atoms or produced artificially.
proton	A positively charged high-energy hydrogen ion with a mass of 1.66 x 10^{-24} g.
Quark	A small subatomic particle inside neutrons and protons.
rad	A unit of absorbed dose equal to 100 ergs/g.
radiation	The emission and propagation of ionizing quanta, particles, or energy through matter or space by atoms or nuclei as a result of radioactive decay or nuclear interactions, as well as electromagnetic radiation.
radiolysis	Decomposition of materials induced by irradiation.
RBE	Relative Biological Effectiveness.

REM   Radiation-equivalent-man. This unit is used for assessment and comparison of biological radiation effects. For example, a radiation dose in a dosimeter could read 1 rad while the person next to the dosimeter could receive 5 REM. In this way, correction factors are applied mathematically to correct for the different responses of biological systems to the various types of penetrating radiation.

Roentgen   The historical unit of exposure

Shielding   The use of material between the radiation source and the point of interest to do one or more of the following:
  o Absorb the radiation.
  o Scatter the radiation away.
  o Degrade the energy through atomic or nuclear interact-actions so it is less effect-ive.

SSC   Superconducting Supercollider.

Sun

Our sun is the source of most of the nuclear energy received by the earth. This solar energy is responsible for life.

threshold

With reference to a radiation damage threshold, the lowest radiation dose which induces permanent change in a measured property (s) of a material; also, the first detectable change in a property of a material due to the effect of radiation.

x-ray

Electromagnetic radiation of frequency between visible light and gamma rays. It may be produced by high energy electrons impinging on a metal target.

INDEX

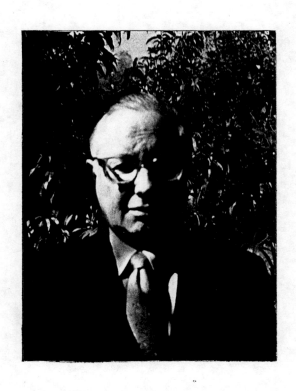

ABOUT THE AUTHOR

Frank L. Bouquet is a physics and engineering
author living in the State of Washington.

After graduating from the University of California at Berkeley, he continued his studies at UCLA.

Over four decades, he worked in various government and industry organizations in the
field of nuclear energy. This book is an out
growth of lectures in Science Seminar and
Fundamentals of Nuclear Radiation that he
taught for six years.